This book is due for return on or before the last date shown below.

D1345261

Don Gresswell Ltd., London, N.21 Cat. No. 1208   DG 02242/71

SMALL ANIMAL PHYSICAL DIAGNOSIS
and Clinical Procedures

SMALL ANIMAL PHYSICAL DIAGNOSIS

and Clinical Procedures

DENNIS M. McCURNIN, D.V.M. , M.S.

Diplomate, American College of Veterinary Surgeons
Professor of Clinical Sciences and Hospital Director
Veterinary Teaching Hospital
College of Veterinary Medicine and Biomedical Sciences
Colorado State University
Fort Collins, Colorado

ELLEN M. POFFENBARGER, D.V.M.

Diplomate, American College of Veterinary Internal Medicine
Assistant Professor of Clinical Sciences
Veterinary Teaching Hospital
College of Veterinary Medicine and Biomedical Sciences
Colorado State University
Fort Collins, Colorado

With 27 full-color illustrations

1991
W.B. SAUNDERS COMPANY *Philadelphia, London, Toronto, Montreal, Sydney, Tokyo*
Harcourt Brace Jovanovich, Inc.

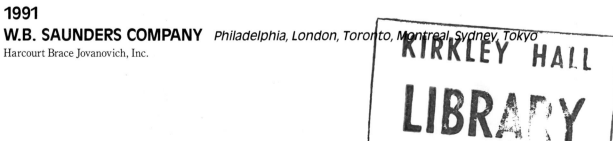

W. B. SAUNDERS COMPANY

Harcourt Brace Jovanovich, Inc.

The Curtis Center
Independence Square West
Philadelphia, PA 19106

Library of Congress Cataloging-in-Publication Data

Small animal physical diagnosis and clinical procedures/[edited by]
  Dennis M. McCurnin, Ellen M. Poffenbarger.
      p.   cm.
    Includes index.
    ISBN 0-7216-5931-4
    1. Dogs — Diseases — Diagnosis.   2. Cats — Diseases — Diagnosis.
      3. Veterinary medicine — Diagnosis, Physical.   4. Veterinary clinical pathology.
      I. McCurnin, Dennis M.   II. Poffenbarger, Ellen M.
    [DNLM: 1. Animal Diseases — diagnosis.   2. Animals, Domestic.
      3. Medical History Taking — veterinary.   4. Physical Examination — veterinary.
      SF 772.5   S635]
    SF991.S595   1991
    636.089'6075 — dc20
    DNLM/DLC   90-8543

Editor: Darlene Pedersen

Developmental Editor: Les Hoeltzel

Designer: Karen O'Keefe

Production Manager: Frank Polizzano

Illustration Coordinator: Matt Andrews

Indexer: Ellen Murray

SMALL ANIMAL PHYSICAL DIAGNOSIS
and Clinical Procedures   ISBN 0-7216-5931-4

Last digit is the print number: 9   8   7   6   5   4   3   2   1

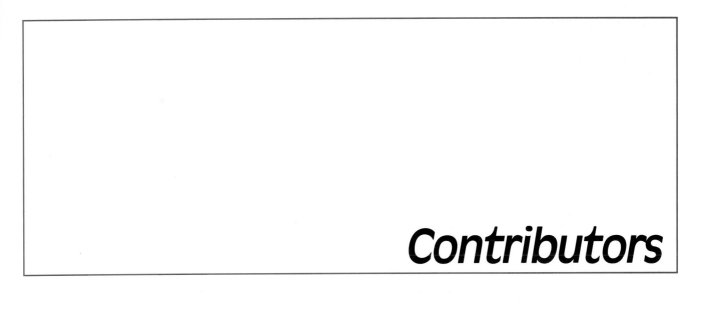

Contributors

BARBARA H. McGUIRE, D.V.M.

Associate Veterinarian, Rio Grande Animal Clinic, Albuquerque, New Mexico

HOWARD B. SEIM III, D.V.M.

Diplomate, American College of Veterinary Surgeons; Associate Professor of Small Animal Surgery, College of Veterinary Medicine and Biomedical Sciences, Colorado State University; Staff Surgeon, Veterinary Teaching Hospital, Fort Collins, Colorado

Preface

Veterinary medicine has truly become a member of the healing professions. The traditional role of our profession has been to care for all animals on the planet. However, we have a broader level of knowledge and understanding now that includes the human-animal bond.

Most of our historical information about our patients must come from the animal owner. Our patients communicate in their own ways to us, but we must also be skilled in obtaining pertinent information from our clients. Accurate historical client information can be as important as the patient's clinical finding.

The complete detailed physical examination is an absolute requirement for each clinical diagnosis. Short cuts taken in the physical examination often mislead the clinician into use of therapeutic and management techniques that are unsuccessful.

An abbreviated physical examination may be the result of an early positive finding in one system or lack of time or interest on the part of the veterinarian. The end result, however, is an incomplete collection of vital clinical data which may result in a misdiagnosis or an incomplete diagnosis.

Small Animal Physical Diagnosis and Clinical Procedures is devoted to the execution of a complete physical examination using the systems approach. Each body system is reviewed in detail, with clinical examples of typical findings provided. Through the systems approach, the total clinical picture can be constructed. Omission of one or more systems in the evaluation process provides an incomplete picture.

The second part of the book presents methods of clinical evaluations. These techniques are outlined in a step-by-step format using clinical illustrations and photographs. The procedures presented are the most commonly used evaluation techniques in a clinical examination.

The techniques offered herein will become the most commonly used skills developed by the clinican. The mastery of these skills and techniques will determine one's clinical success. When physical examination short cuts are used, the quality of patient care is lessened.

The purpose of *Small Animal Physical Diagnosis and Clinical Procedures* is to provide veterinary medical students and veterinary technician students with a system-by-system approach to a complete physical examination. An early commitment and understanding of the value of a complete physical examination will help provide a lifetime of quality patient care.

DENNIS M. MCCURNIN, D.V.M.
BATON ROUGE, LOUISIANA

Contents

27 *Full-color ILLUSTRATIONS*

Contents **x**

PART

1

PHYSICAL DIAGNOSIS and HISTORY TAKING

Philosophy of Physical Diagnosis and History Taking

ELLEN M. POFFENBARGER

The principal obligation of the veterinarian to her client* and patient is the establishment of a diagnosis and institution of therapy, if necessary, for each animal that is examined. Diagnosis involves collecting data about the pet by a variety of means and then analyzing the data so as to propose a hypothesis regarding the cause of the patient's problem(s). Diagnosis requires a basic knowledge of medicine acquired by standard medical education and experience, inference based on that knowledge, and the selection of diagnostic tests, which include the history and physical examination as well as laboratory, radiographic, or other procedures. The history and physical examination may be the only sources of information needed for the diagnosis or may provide data useful in determining the most appropriate diagnostic tests to be performed.

A carefully taken history of the pet's problem should be the initial diagnostic step in each animal examined. An example of the benefits of a complete history follows.

> On her way to work, an owner drops her dog off at 7:30 A.M. for her veterinarian to examine because she says the dog has been vomiting for 3 days. During the day, laboratory tests including a complete blood count, serum chemistry panel, urinalysis, and abdominal radiographs fail to establish a diagnosis of the problem. When the owner picks up the dog that afternoon, she is upset that no diagnosis has been made. Upon questioning the owner about the vomiting, the veterinarian finds out that the dog is bringing up food within 30 minutes of eating. The food appears undigested, is cylindrical in shape, and comes up without effort on the dog's part. It is now apparent that the dog has not been vomiting but has been regurgitating. An explanation is now necessary as to why chest radiographs are indicated to look at the esophagus instead of the abdominal radiographs

---

*The pronoun "she" is used throughout to refer to both client and veterinarian.

that were already taken. Taking the time initially to question the owner would have saved time, money, and embarrassment.

Diagnostic tests cannot replace the information to be gained from a complete history and physical examination. The tests in the example above were chosen because it was thought the dog was vomiting as a result of an abnormality in the stomach, intestinal tract, or other organ system that can secondarily cause vomiting (kidneys, liver, pancreas). These tests were inappropriate and unrewarding in the diagnosis of an esophageal problem.

The physical examination of a pet is essential to diagnosis of the pet's problem. Normal as well as abnormal findings can be very helpful in the diagnostic process. The case example above can be expanded to illustrate this point.

A thorough physical examination was completed and revealed distention of the neck to the left of the trachea near the thoracic inlet. In addition, gurgling noises could be auscultated in this area. Upon examination of the oral cavity, pooling of saliva and food was evident in the oropharynx, and the dog had a reduced gag reflex. The dog was bright, alert, and in good condition. There were no other abnormalities found on physical examination. These findings are consistent with a megaesophagus and, in spite of the lack of an accurate history, should make an astute veterinarian suspicious of an esophageal problem.

The practice of medicine is imprecise. Consequently, there is an artistic as well as a scientific component. Its principal and distinctive feature is human ability.[1] What elements of human ability, then, are necessary for a good doctor to refine? The foremost is the power of *attention,* the concentration of the mind on a single thought or object (the owner of the animal during the history taking or the animal during the physical examination). This sounds simple, but very few professionals ever attain it. Attention is an active process, one that requires continual conscious thought. A carefully performed history and physical examination can be used together to initiate an appropriate and logical sequence leading to a diagnosis. They complement each other and can be used in conjunction with laboratory and radiographic data. No one source of information should stand alone in the determination of a diagnosis.

The physical diagnosis section of *Small Animal Physical Diagnosis and Clinical Procedures* is to be used as a guide for veterinary students and veterinary technicians to the art of history taking and physical examination. It is hoped that it will be a valuable source of basic techniques that are helpful in gathering information about the patient. It may serve as a reference to graduate veterinarians who wish to refresh their skills in this area. This section provides examples of methods of information gathering. Common abnormal findings are illustrated for each system examined. This section is not a comprehensive volume of all possible outcomes, however.

The objectives of this section are as follows:

1. To provide the veterinary student and technician who are just beginning to learn about the art of veterinary medicine with basic methods of collecting information about the patient
2. To provide a guide to interviewing clients to maximize the quantity and quality of information gained
3. To provide a source of basic examination techniques and common abnormalities that might be observed when examining the various body systems

REFERENCES

1. Wyngaarden JB, Smith LH Jr (eds): Cecil Textbook of Medicine, 17th ed. Philadelphia, WB Saunders, 1985.

RECOMMENDED READING

1. Bates B: A Guide to Physical Diagnosis and History Taking, 4th ed. Philadelphia, JB Lippincott, 1987.
2. Hardy RM: General physical examination of the canine patient. Vet Clin North Am 11(3):453–467, 1981.
3. Harvey AM, Bordley J, Barondess JA: Differential Diagnosis: The Interpretation of Clinical Evidence, 3rd ed. Philadelphia, WB Saunders, 1979.
4. Wyngaarden JB, Smith LH Jr (eds): Cecil Textbook of Medicine, 18th ed. Philadelphia, WB Saunders, 1988.

The Health History

As you begin to talk with clients about their pets, several things begin to happen. You *collect information* necessary to form an initial problem list for that animal. You *initiate a relationship* with the client and her pet which, it is hoped, helps them to learn to trust and confide in you. You also begin to *share knowledge* with the client about her pet, which leads to a better understanding of the pet's problems. *Problems are initially defined* during the health history, which forms a basis for *formulating diagnostic and therapeutic plans.*

OVERVIEW OF THE HISTORY-TAKING PROCESS

The history of an animal should include the following:

1. Date of examination
2. Signalment (client and patient identification)
3. Chief complaint
4. History of the present illness
5. Past medical history
6. Current health status
7. Systems review

The specifics of these seven components are discussed later in this chapter. In addition to these, a complete medical history should also contain the following:

1. Family medical history (health of sire, dam, littermates)
2. Vaccination history
3. Travel history
4. Diet history
5. Environmental history
6. Birth history (if less than 6 months old)

Meeting the Client and Patient

Before beginning the interview process, greet the client by his or her appropriate title (Mr., Miss, Mrs., Ms., Dr.) and call the pet by name. Introduce yourself and briefly explain the procedures to follow. The actual interview may then begin. The most important attribute that a veterinarian or technician can have is the ability to *listen*. Effective listening often provides the diagnostic edge needed to resolve a difficult clinical problem. A calm, unhurried attitude projects an image of sensitivity to the client.

It is often helpful to let the client describe the problem in her own way initially. In this way, the client feels that you are really trying to understand her pet's problem. Often, if you begin the questioning first, the client does not understand how the questions asked relate to the animal's problem. She can become angry and frustrated that you are not listening to her. It is important to take notes as the client speaks so they may be referred to later.

Questioning the Client

After the client explains what she perceives to be the problem, additional questions can be asked to clarify the abnormalities. Start with general questions and proceed to the more specific. For example, if an animal is presented for a problem of diarrhea, it may be helpful to know if the stool is loose or if the frequency of bowel movements has changed. Following this, it may be important to know how many times a day the animal has a bowel movement, whether the animal is straining or not, and the character of the stool. Questions should be asked in such a way as to be unbiased. In other words, ask questions that do not imply a particular response, for example, "Does your cat go to the litter box more frequently?" versus "Have there been any changes in the urinary habits of your cat?" A client who likes to be agreeable will answer the first question "Yes" because it sounds like the interviewer expects the cat to be going to the litter box more frequently, not necessarily because her cat *is* going to the litter box more frequently. There is no bias in the second phrasing of the question.

Accurate information can be better obtained by asking questions that require a graded response rather than a yes or no answer. For example, if a dog is presented for examination because it collapses after exercise, you may ask, "How far do you walk with your pet before he collapses?" instead of "Does your dog seem to tire and collapse quickly?" Multiple-choice questions may also be helpful in obtaining the desired information.

During the interview, ask only one question at a time. Let the client answer the question as best she can before asking another question. Direct eye contact should be made with the client as frequently as possible. This provides a clear message that her problem is being dealt with on a high priority level. Written notes should be made in the medical record while facing the client.

It is sometimes difficult to differentiate client observations about her pet from her conclusions. Since most of our clients have no medical training, their conclusions are sometimes erroneous. But their powers of observation of their pet may be remarkable. An example of this follows.

> An older man brings his cat to the clinic with the complaint that the cat is constipated. If left at that, one might send the cat home on stool softeners. Upon further clarification of the problem, the man thinks his cat is constipated because he has observed the cat going to the litter box frequently and straining but producing no feces. A physical examination reveals that the cat's bladder is the size of a handball and rock hard. The history and physical examination suggest that the cat has a urethral obstruction that could result in a life-threatening situation if not resolved rapidly.

During an interview, do not be afraid to repeat a question or rephrase the question to clarify the problem. In addition, it is not uncommon to obtain subsequent history over the phone or in person if it might help the overall understanding of the case.

It is important to use terms the client can understand. The level of knowledge is quite diverse among clients; therefore, one may have to speak in simple terms to some clients, whereas others may understand medical terminology completely. A question like "Have your dog's defecation habits changed?" may evoke a negative response when in fact the owner did not understand the question but said "No" to avoid being embarrassed. Therefore, you must be assured that you and the client are talking about the same thing.

As in any interview process, the source of the information must be taken into consideration when interpreting the data. Is the information reliable? Often in veterinary medicine, people other than the owner present the animal for examination. It may be the neighbor who really does not observe the animal regularly, or it may be a child who does not understand the animal's problem or the questions asked. If at all possible, the person closest to the animal should be present to answer questions when the animal is examined.

Feelings of guilt regarding the pet may result in an unsatisfactory interview. For example, intentional or unintentional trauma to the animal or possible ingestion by the pet of an illegal drug may be reasons that the client does not reveal the whole truth. The client's trust, then, becomes important in bringing out the necessary information.

A common problem in veterinary medicine is the inability of the owner to observe the animal. If an owner of a strictly outdoor cat is asked "Does the cat vomit?", the response may be "No" when in fact the real answer to the question should be "I have never seen my cat vomit but my opportunities to observe her are few." Probably the question would have been better phrased, "Do you observe your cat frequently enough to know if she is vomiting or not?"

Several special client-related problems may interfere with a particular client's ability to relay information. For people who by nature are quiet, good communication skills are required to gain the needed information. Active listening can help in this situation. Prompting the person with phrases such as "Go on," or "Tell me what you mean by . . ." can often lead her to explain things in more detail. Some clients are at the other extreme and talk too much. The veterinarian and technician must develop ways to draw out information from some clients and to encourage other clients to move on to the next important piece of information. Older pets with multiple problems can create difficulty in gaining clear-cut information on each indi-

Colorado State University

Veterinary Teaching Hospital
Fort Collins, Colorado 80523

HISTORY

HOSPITAL REGULATION: ALL POSITIVE AS WELL AS NEGATIVE FINDINGS SHALL BE RECORDED

DATE _____ HOUR _____ [A.M.] [P.M.]

ORDER
OF
RECORDING

1. (CC) CHIEF
   COMPLAINT
2. (HPI) HISTORY
   OF PRESENT ILLNESS
3. (PH) PAST
   HISTORY
   A. MEDICAL
   B. SURGICAL
   C. TRAUMA
   D. VACCINATIONS
   E. COGGINS
   F. WORMING
4. (EH) ENVIRONMENTAL
   HISTORY
5. INSURANCE
6. (SR) SYSTEM
   REVIEW
   A. GENERAL
   B. SKIN
   C. HEAD/NECK
   D. (EENT) EYES-EARS-
      NOSE-THROAT
   E. RESPIRATORY
   F. CARDIOVASCULAR
   G. (GI) GASTRO-
      INTESTINAL
   H. URINARY
   I. REPRODUCTIVE
   J. MUSCULOSKELETAL
   K. NERVOUS
7. SIGNATURE

ATTENDING CLINICIAN

MR 125 Rev. 2/87   HISTORY

Figure 2–1. A preprinted form will aid in the accurate recording of the history. (With permission of the Colorado State University Veterinary Teaching Hospital, Fort Collins, CO.)

vidual problem from owners who are confused and upset about their pets.

Angry or hostile clients hinder a relationship. A client may be angry at previous veterinarians who have failed to diagnose and/or effectively treat her pet's problem. The owner of an ill pet may be feeling the anger of futility or the realization of her pet's impending death. The sadness associated with a pet's death may result in the inability of the owner to answer questions without crying.

Some owners may not be able to understand questions well enough to answer them. Language barriers, including deafness or a foreign language, can also hinder the acquisition of a good history. These problems can lead to considerable difficulties in communication; however, a little time and effort can usually overcome most of them.

After all the information on the chief complaint has been collected, it is best to summarize the problems for the client. In this way, any misunderstandings about the pet's problem may be perceived and corrected.

Accurate recording of the history is just as important as taking the history. The history may be recorded on a form designed for this purpose, which can become a permanent part of the animal's record (Fig. 2–1). This reduces confusion, saves time during future visits, and provides background for other veterinarians who may examine the pet.

CONTENT OF A COMPREHENSIVE HISTORY

Signalment

The signalment of the animal includes the age, breed, and sex. It should be the first information about the pet that is requested. Age is important in that different subsets of disease affect animals of various ages with different frequencies. Young animals are more likely to present with illnesses caused by infectious organisms, toxins, foreign bodies, and parasites, whereas older animals present most often with diseases caused by degenerative processes or neoplasia. Certain breeds of dogs or cats have hereditary predispositions to certain diseases; therefore, just knowing the breed brings to mind possible causes for the animal's problem. For example, cervical vertebral instability is more likely in a Doberman pinscher with posterior paresis, but a dachshund may have similar signs due to a ruptured thoracolumbar intervertebral disc. The sex of the animal also helps narrow the diagnostic possibilities. For instance, pyometra can be a cause of increased thirst and urination (polyuria/polydipsia) in an intact female dog but need not be included in the list of differential diagnoses for polyuria/polydipsia in a male dog.

Chief Complaint

The chief complaint is the reason that the owner has presented the animal for examination. It is the *most important* thing on her mind, and it should be the first matter of discussion. As mentioned above, letting the owner discuss the problem as she sees it is often the best way to obtain the information needed. Facilitate the discussion with cues such as "I'm listening." Questions may be asked as needed to clarify the problem.

History of the Present Illness

The history of the present illness is obtained by a series of questions regarding the chief complaint, which seek to characterize the problem. The more that is known about the problem, the more the diagnostic possibilities may be narrowed down. Questions asked should pertain to the location, quality, severity, onset, duration, frequency, setting, factors that increase or decrease the signs, associated problems, and progression or improvement of the problem. Not all of these questions are easily applied to all problems, but as many of them as possible should be answered. Two examples follow.

> Patient 1, a 3-year-old spayed female poodle, is presented because of a cough. The cough is characterized as honking (quality). The owner says that the dog has episodes of coughing that seem to "wear her out" (severity). The cough began 2 weeks ago (onset), and she has been coughing ever since (duration). She has coughing spells 6 to 8 times a day (frequency). Excitement, such as the doorbell ringing, seems to initiate the episodes (setting). At rest, she seems perfectly fine (factors that decrease the signs). Her tongue turns blue and she collapses at the end of some episodes (associated manifestations). It seems to be getting worse with time (progression).

> This history and signalment are consistent with a diagnosis of tracheal collapse, although other things may cause similar signs.

> Patient 2, a 12-year-old neutered male domestic short-hair cat, is brought in with a complaint of a lump under his jaw. The lump is in the area of the angle of the mandible on the right side (location). The owner says it is a hard structure that drains bloody fluid occasionally (quality). It seems to bother the cat because he won't eat (severity). The owner noticed it 1 week ago (onset). There was no injury in that area as far as the owner knows (setting). The owner says that he has tried to put warm compresses on the area but there has been no change (factors that may increase or decrease the signs). The cat paws at the mass sometimes (associated manifestations). The mass seems to have grown in the past week (progression).

> In a cat of this age, neoplasia is the most likely cause of the cat's problem; however, abscess or granuloma may look similar.

Characterization of the problem permits one to make informed decisions regarding the need for diagnostic tests and therapeutic intervention. The information in the above case examples may have been obtained from the owner during his own description of the complaint or prompted by questions from the veterinarian. How the information is obtained is not as important as the content of the information. Two different cases follow to illustrate this point.

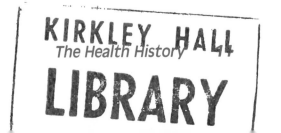

Patient 3, a 9-year-old spayed female poodle, is presented with a complaint of coughing. The cough sounds moist to the owner (quality). The cough began 1 month ago (onset), but it does not seem to bother the dog at all (severity). She coughs four to five times in a 24-hour period (frequency), and the frequency is increasing (progression). The coughing seems to be worse at night but also occurs during the day when the dog is resting (setting). She seems to be more "tired" than when she was younger (associated manifestations).

The signalment and description of the cough in this dog suggest that the cough may be related to cardiac disease, possible congestive heart failure.

Patient 4, a 2-year-old intact male cat, is presented for examination because of a lump over the tailhead region. The lump is just to the right of the tailhead (location). It is a soft mass (quality) and the cat seems very pained when the lump is touched (severity). The owner just noticed it this morning (onset), but the cat was out last night (setting). If you raise his tail, the cat screams in pain (factors that increase the signs). He would not eat this morning either (associated manifestations).

A painful lump in this area on a young adult male cat is suggestive of an abscess.

Patients 3 and 4 have the same chief complaints as Patients 1 and 2, respectively. From the more detailed history, it is easy to list possible causes that are more likely than others. The location of the problem focuses one's mind on a specific set of disease processes that commonly occur in the affected area. The quality of the sign helps characterize the problem better and may aid in localization. For example, diarrhea can be localized to the large or small bowel based on several qualities (Table 2–1).

Table 2–1 LOCALIZATION OF THE CAUSE OF DIARRHEA		
Quality	**Large Bowel**	**Small Bowel**
Mucus	Yes	No
Fresh blood	Yes	No
Frequency	Increased	Normal
Amount	Small	Normal to increased
Form	Loose to formed	No form, watery

The severity of the disease aids in the decision to do diagnostic tests immediately (life-threatening illness) or to wait to see if the problem is going to persist (minor problem). Additionally, therapeutic measures may need to be instituted immediately in a severely ill animal.

A time/sign graph is useful in interpreting the onset, duration, and progression of an illness (Fig. 2–2). Infectious or traumatic diseases have an acute onset, rapid development of clinical signs, and rapid or gradual improvement with appropriate therapy. Degenerative or

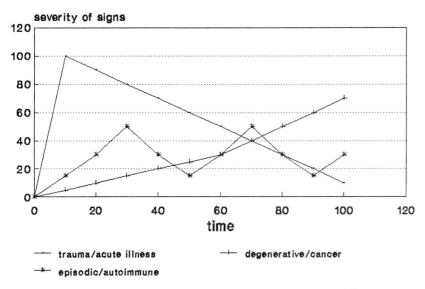

severity of signs

— trauma/acute illness   + degenerate/cancer
-*- episodic/autoimmune

Figure 2-2. A time/sign graph will help to define the etiology of disease processes.

neoplastic diseases, on the other hand, often have an insidious onset and become progressively worse with time. If the sign is recurrent or episodic, the frequency may again help define the significance of the problem and indicate whether diagnostic tests are necessary.

The setting in which the problem occurs can also provide clues to what illness the animal may have, as illustrated in the examples above. The 3-year-old poodle that coughs on excitement is more likely to have tracheal collapse than is the 9-year-old poodle that coughs at night (more consistent with congestive heart failure). Prior treatment or environmental conditions that increase or decrease the clinical signs are important. For instance, a dog that is seen for episodic weakness, vomiting, and depression has responded to cortisone injections by another veterinarian in the past but the problem has been recurrent. This history should suggest hypoadrenocorticism as a possible cause of the dog's problems. Associated disease manifestations can also help narrow the diagnostic possibilities. For example, diarrhea associated with weight loss, anorexia, and occasional vomiting is more likely to be of small bowel origin than large. Therefore, only diseases of the small bowel need be considered when initiating a diagnostic work-up.

Past Medical History

The importance of the past medical history cannot be underestimated. This information includes puppy or kitten diseases, adult illnesses, traumatic injuries, and previous surgeries. Any of these items may alter the approach to the patient both diagnostically and therapeutically. For example, a draining tract on the leg of a cat that had a surgically corrected fracture at that site most likely is a problem related to that surgery. A dog with a previous diagnosis of chronic renal failure is not a good candidate for gentamicin therapy for a respiratory infection, because gentamicin is nephrotoxic. A dog with a history of hypoadrenocorticism that arrives in a state of hypovolemic shock should be treated as if it is in a hypoadrenal crisis. The list of examples could go on, but suffice it to say that a complete and accurate history is crucial if the animal is to be managed properly.

Current Health Status

The current health status describes the animal's present condition with respect to several areas of interest. The date of the last *vaccination* provides information on the animal's level of protection against the common infectious diseases. This is especially important in the young animal. Also included in this topic is the type of *environment* the animal lives in. Is it an indoor or outdoor pet? This information determines the potential for exposure to infectious disease, trauma, and poisons. Is there a fenced-in yard or does the dog run free (potential for trauma or poisoning)? If an outdoor animal, is there protection for the animal from the weather (heat or cold exposure)? Is there access to garbage or stored chemicals (potential for toxicity or foreign object ingestion)? The *diet* of the animal, including the type of food and the quantity, should not be overlooked, especially if the animal has a problem related to the gastrointestinal tract. The amount and type of *exercise* the animal receives provide insight into obesity, orthopedic problems, and so forth. Questions regarding *current medications* (type, dose, frequency) allow continued medication of the animal should it be hospitalized and help avoid the prescription of drugs incompatible with each other.

The *travel history* and *family history* may provide insight into the probability of certain differential diagnoses. Although specific diseases may not be prevalent in one area of the country, pets travel with their families and may be exposed to diseases uncommon in their particular home region. Heartworm disease, blastomycosis, coccidioidomycosis, Lyme disease, and Rocky Mountain spotted fever are a few examples of regional diseases. Although family history is difficult to obtain on most animals, it can be a source of important information if available. In very young animals with clinical signs suggestive of an infectious disease, it is helpful to know if other littermates are ill. In the case of heritable defects, knowledge of littermates with the suspected disease helps support the diagnosis.

Systems Review

The systems review section of the history-taking process is an attempt to gain information about problems other than the chief complaint. In this portion of the interview, two or three key questions are asked regarding each of the major body systems. These questions are designed to detect problems related or unrelated to the chief complaint. For instance, a dog is presented with a complaint of persistent fever. This problem by itself is not helpful in localizing its cause. However, when asked about the respiratory system, the owner replies that the dog also has had a cough. The cough helps to localize the problem to the respiratory tract, which is likely the source of the fever. This avenue should be pursued first before the many other causes of fever are explored. In addition, many patients have more than one problem. The work-up of an animal with multiple problems can be complicated and expensive. Making the owner aware of this early on can avoid misunderstandings later. Communication gaps are the leading cause of malpractice claims against veterinarians.

Sample Questions for a Review of the Systems

A. **General.** Has there been any change in the weight of your pet? Has your animal had a fever?

B. **Integument.** Has there been any hair loss? Does your pet scratch or chew at itself excessively? Are there any rashes, bumps, or sores?

C. **Head/neck.** Are there any abnormal swellings in this area? How is the head carried? What is the animal's attitude like?

D. **Ears/eyes/nose/throat.** Is there any discharge from the ears or eyes? Does the animal seem to see all right? Does the animal respond to noises? Has there been any change in the voice?

E. **Respiratory.** Has there been any coughing or sneezing? Does the animal seem to breathe normally?

F. **Cardiovascular.** Does your pet cough? Does your pet exercise the same as before?

G. **Gastrointestinal.** Has there been any vomiting or diarrhea? How is your pet's appetite?

H. **Genitourinary.** Has there been any change in your pet's urinary habits? Is your pet spayed/neutered? If so, when? If not, any litters produced? Any vaginal or preputial discharge? Excessive licking of the genital area?

I. **Musculoskeletal.** Does your pet exhibit any weakness? Does your pet favor any leg when it walks or runs?

J. **Nervous.** What is your pet's general attitude like? Is your pet able to walk normally? Does your pet seem weak? Has your pet ever had seizures?

RECOMMENDED READING

1. Bates B: A Guide to Physical Examination and History Taking, 4th ed. Philadelphia, JB Lippincott, 1987.
2. Harvey AM, Bordley J, Barondess JA: Differential Diagnosis: The Interpretation of Clinical Evidence, 3rd ed. Philadelphia, WB Saunders, 1979.

The Physical Examination as a Diagnostic Tool

The physical examination in combination with the health history can be the key to the diagnosis of a patient's problem. Veterinarians and technicians must both show a **sensitivity** toward the animal to gain the animal's as well as the owner's trust. The sensitivity shown toward the animal and the client can determine the amount of information one is able to get from the physical examination as well as whether the client will return in the future. It is important to move slowly, palpate gently, and talk to the animal and owner about what is being done and why. Rushing an examination not only may result in missing problems but may make the animal fearful and uncooperative.

Attentiveness is of paramount importance. As each system is examined, a multitude of observations are made. Normal findings are seldom registered consciously. It is the abnormal information that must be stored and recalled later. It is not uncommon to perform a physical examination without directing full attention to the patient. The owner may be talking or one may be concerned about another patient that is not doing well. The power of observation is one's strongest asset if it is utilized. **Completeness** of the examination process is an important objective. Mistakes are more frequently caused by failure to observe or register an abnormality than by not knowing the significance of that abnormality. Discontinuing an examination at the point of finding one abnormality is a common mistake. Multiple abnormalities are often found when a complete examination is performed.

During the physical examination, several senses can be utilized. The most valuable senses during the physical examination are **sight** and **touch.** Animals can be observed from a distance initially, then more closely for defects in symmetry, gait, posture, and attitude. The sense of touch is important in detecting abnormalities that may be hidden beneath a thick coat of fur or inside an abdomen. Abnormal odors may be detected by the sense of **smell** and can be indicators of specific disease. For example, ketotic diabetics may have a sweet odor of ketones to their breath. The sense of **hearing** is especially important during auscultation of the chest but may be important in detecting a voice change and abnormal intestinal sounds as well.

Methods of Information Gathering

There are four means of information gathering during a complete physical examination. The first is **observation.** Hundreds of observations are made during a physical examination, and concentration on the abnormal findings is essential. **Palpation** is the second tool of the examiner. Palpation is defined in *Dorland's Illustrated Medical Dictionary* as "the application of the fingers with light pressure to the surface of the body for the purpose of determining the consistency of the parts beneath." Palpation has a wide variety of applications in the physical examination process; these are discussed in detail under examination of specific systems. A third means of information collection is **auscultation,** or "the act of listening for sounds within the body, chiefly for ascertaining the condition of the lungs, heart, pleura, abdomen, and other organs, and for the detection of pregnancy." Although a trained ear may be able to hear some sounds, a stethoscope is the necessary instrument for this mode of examination. Fourth, **percussion** can provide information regarding certain conditions. Percussion is "the act of striking a part with short, sharp blows as an aid in diagnosing the condition of the underlying parts by the sound obtained." To perform percussion, the middle finger of one hand is placed on the area to be percussed and the flexed middle finger of the other hand is used to strike that finger. The tapping initiates a vibration that is perceived as a sound dependent on the physical characteristics of the tissues beneath. Pleural effusion, pulmonary consolidation, and intrathoracic masses may dampen the normal sounds heard when percussing the chest. Pneumothorax or emphysema may result in a hyper-resonant sound.

Recording the Findings

The physical examination findings must be recorded in a concise, logical manner. Proper recording of physical abnormalities is important in planning the diagnostic tests to be performed as well as in planning for therapy. In busy practices, it is impossible to remember all the problems of all the different animals seen in one day, let alone a week or month. Since it is now common in veterinary practice to have multidoctor hospitals in which the same veterinarian may not see the animal each time, the recorded data are critical to quality care of the patient. The medical record serves as a basis for future comparison if the animal returns with the same or new problems. A complete and clearly written medical record is the only legal evidence in cases involving litigation. The documentation of the physical examination is of crucial importance.

An efficient method of recording data accurately is a physical examination form that becomes a permanent part of the animal's record (Fig. 3–1). It can be combined with the history form described in Chapter 2. The physical examination form lists body systems with boxes to check if the system is normal or abnormal. There is space on the page for details about those systems that are determined to be abnormal. In addition, standard information about the animal (name of the pet and owner, signalment of the pet, address of the owner), body weight, temperature, pulse rate, and respiration rate can be recorded.

Sources of Errors

Given all that is involved in performing a physical examination and recording the data, there is always the possibility of errors. Errors

---

PHYSICAL EXAMINATION

(1) GENERAL APPEARANCE ☐ Normal ☐ Abnormal	(2) INTEGUMENTARY ☐ Normal ☐ Abnormal ☐ Not examined	(3) MUSCULOSKELETAL ☐ Normal ☐ Abnormal ☐ Not examined	(4) CIRCULATORY ☐ Normal ☐ Abnormal ☐ Not examined
(5) RESPIRATORY ☐ Normal ☐ Abnormal ☐ Not examined	(6) DIGESTIVE ☐ Normal ☐ Abnormal ☐ Not examined	(7) GENITOURINARY ☐ Normal ☐ Abnormal ☐ Not examined	(8) EYES ☐ Normal ☐ Abnormal ☐ Not examined
(9) EARS ☐ Normal ☐ Abnormal ☐ Not examined	(10) NEURAL SYSTEM ☐ Normal ☐ Abnormal ☐ Not examined	(11) LYMPH NODES ☐ Normal ☐ Abnormal ☐ Not examined	(12) MUCOUS MEMBRANES ☐ Normal ☐ Abnormal ☐ Not examined

DESCRIBE ABNORMAL: (Use numbers above) T _____ P _____ R _____ Wt. _____ ☐ SCALE ☐ EST.

LESION LOCATION

VIEW

DORSAL ☐   VENTRAL ☐

PRINTED STUDENT NAME   CLINICIAN SIGNATURE

SIZE _____

TEMPORARY PROBLEM LIST	DIFFERENTIAL DIAGNOSES	DIAGNOSTIC PLAN	THERAPEUTIC PLAN
(1)			
(2)			
(3)			

MR 125 Rev. 1/85

Figure 3–1. A physical examination form lends itself to easy recording of data and filing in the patient's permanent record. (With permission of the Colorado State University Veterinary Teaching Hospital, Fort Collins, CO.)

may be categorized as those of omission, technique, detection, interpretation, and recording.[1] An error of omission is made when the examiner fails to examine a part or system. Using a physical examination form can minimize this type of error. Inexperience and lack of patient cooperation are responsible for errors in technique. These include disorganized examination, improper use of instruments, and poor bedside manner (causing patient discomfort or hostility). In addition, faulty or missing equipment is included in this type of error. Errors in detection involve overlooking an abnormality that is present, reporting an abnormality that is not present, and interpreting a normal anatomic or physiologic finding as abnormal. Failure to understand the importance of an abnormal finding and lack of knowledge regarding the value of an abnormal finding in the diagnostic process are considered errors of interpretation. Recording errors include illegible handwriting, failure to record an abnormal finding, recording a finding that was not present, using obscure abbreviations, improper terminology, and incomplete recording of a diagnosis. Attentiveness and careful record keeping minimize mistakes.

Getting Ready for the Examination

Optimal environmental conditions improve the data obtained when doing a physical examination. Use a quiet room with no distractions. Adequate lighting is a necessity. Awkward positions for the examiner or the pet hinder the examination; therefore, all but the largest dogs should be examined on a table that brings the animal to a comfortable height. This also inhibits the animal's attempts to escape so that more time can be spent looking at the animal and less time chasing it.

When approaching the animal for the first time it is important to socialize with it. Approach the animal slowly and offer the animal a hand to sniff. (If aggressiveness is detected, this step may be omitted.) Allow the animal time to get to know you. Often it is worthwhile to pet and talk to the animal while obtaining the history. Animals express many different emotions at the veterinary office, ranging from fear to excitement to rolling over on their backs for a rub on the tummy. It is a distinct advantage to be able to complete the physical examination with the animal as calm as possible.

In most instances, restraint for the physical examination process is easily provided by the owner or a technician. Often, all that is necessary is to place the animal on the examining table and have the owner talk to the animal and gently hold the head. Large breed dogs can be examined on the floor with the owner holding the collar or leash to steady the animal. In the case of the pampered pet who wants to climb on the owner's shoulder continuously, it is wise to have another person restrain the animal. The aggressive animal is difficult to examine completely. A muzzle should be applied to an aggressive dog to protect the veterinarian, technician, and owner, but this limits the ability to examine the oral cavity. In addition, it may make the animal more fractious and the struggling that results prohibits further examination. An aggressive cat can be worse than an aggressive dog. When attempts to socialize the cat have failed, a towel over the head may calm the cat enough to allow the examination. In extreme instances, tranquilization of the cat or dog may be necessary to complete a physical examination, realizing that some parameters (heart rate, respiratory rate, body temperature, and neurologic parameters) will be altered by the drug.

Very little equipment is needed to do a physical examination. A light source such as a penlight is helpful for examining the eyes, ears, and mouth. An otoophthalmoscope is beneficial but not necessary for a general examination. Auscultation of the thorax requires a good quality stethoscope that feels comfortable. A rectal thermometer to determine the pet's temperature is essential. A pleximeter or reflex hammer aids in the differentiation of neurologic problems. A hemostat is desirable for the determination of sensory function.

A physical examination routine should be developed that can be applied to all patients. The specifics of the routine are not important, but a complete examination of all systems must be accomplished. Many veterinarians start at the animal's nose and work their way back to the tail, examining all areas in between. Others take a different approach by examining systems of the body, such as head and neck, respiratory, cardiovascular, and so on. Sometimes it is convenient to take the systems review portion of the history at the same time the physical examination of that system is being performed. There are probably as many ways to complete a physical examination as there are veterinarians. If a routine is developed, however, consistency in the examination process is gained and there is less likelihood of errors of omission.

In the chapters that follow, the examination of separate systems is discussed. Each system is covered in detail. In the actual physical examination, of course, evaluations of separate systems may be combined. For instance, it is common to auscultate the lungs and heart during the same portion of the examination. Although each is focused on separately, it is not necessary to complete the evaluation of the entire respiratory tract before starting the cardiovascular examination.

The keys to quality physical examination skills are patience, perseverance, and practice.[2] Patience with yourself and with the patient maximizes the information gained from the physical examination. It is important not to give up on developing these skills even though the effort seems unrewarding and frustrating at first. Practicing physical examination techniques on normal animals helps familiarize one with the broad range of normal findings so that one can better identify the abnormal.

THE COMPREHENSIVE PHYSICAL EXAMINATION

The remainder of this section of the book describes the specific physical examination techniques as they apply to various systems of the body. In addition, special considerations regarding the examination of cats are covered at the end of each chapter.

The physical examination begins as you observe the animal in the waiting room. How is the animal interacting with this strange environment? Is the animal alert and responding to all the stimuli surrounding it? Does the animal seem aggressive to other animals or people? Is the animal so ill that it is unaware of or uninterested in its environment? Are there indications of pain, anxiety, or dyspnea?

From a distance, the gait and posture of the animal should be noted as the animal is walked to the examination room. What is the stature of the animal? Achondroplastic breeds may being to mind a certain set of common problems such as stenotic nares, elongated soft palate, and hypoplastic trachea. Is the animal able to ambulate normally? Is there a head tilt? Does the animal limp? Body symmetry or lack thereof should also be noted. Is the animal over- or underweight?

As the history is taken, it is wise to continue to observe the dog or cat for any abnormal traits. After the history is completed, the main part of the physical examination process is begun. The animal should be weighed and the body temperature, pulse rate, and respiratory rate taken.

REFERENCES

1. Hardy RM: General physical examination of the canine patient. Vet Clin North Am 11(3):453–467, 1981.
2. Wiener S, Nathanson M: Physical examination: Frequently observed errors. JAMA 236:852, 1976.

RECOMMENDED READING

1. Bates B: A Guide to Physical Diagnosis and History Taking, 4th ed. Philadelphia, JB Lippincott, 1987.
2. *Dorland's Illustrated Medical Dictionary,* 27th ed. Philadelphia, WB Saunders, 1988.

Head and Neck

APPLIED ANATOMY

Regions of the head take their names from the underlying bones (such as frontal area, occipital area) (Fig. 4–1). This is important in localizing and describing physical examination findings.

The **nose** consists of external and internal portions. The external portion can be examined easily and is composed of the planum nasale, associated cartilages and bones, the nostrils, and the overlying integument. The internal nose consists of the turbinates and that part of the skull in which they are housed.

The **eye and periocular structures** are illustrated in Figure 4–2. The dorsal and ventral palpebrae converge at the medial and lateral canthi. The space between them is the palpebral fissure. Eyelashes or cilia are present along the edge of the upper eyelid. The eyelids are lined with a mucous membrane, the palpebral conjunctiva. This membrane is continued onto the eyeball as the bulbar conjunctiva. The third eyelid, or *nictitating membrane,* is located in the medial canthus of the eye. It may or may not be pigmented. A **T**-shaped cartilage surrounded by the gland of the third eyelid is present within the third eyelid. The visible part of the eyeball is covered by the *sclera* and *cornea.* The sclera covers about 85 per cent of the eye and is white in color. The anterior portion of the eye is the transparent cornea, through which the iris and pupil can be seen. The dog's pupil is normally round. The lens is transparent and biconvex. It separates the anterior and posterior chambers of the eye. The lacrimal gland is located within the periorbital connective tissue in the dorsolateral aspect of the orbit. The lacrimal fluid that lubricates and protects the eyes drains into the puncta and the nasolacrimal duct to empty into the nasal cavity (Fig. 4–3).

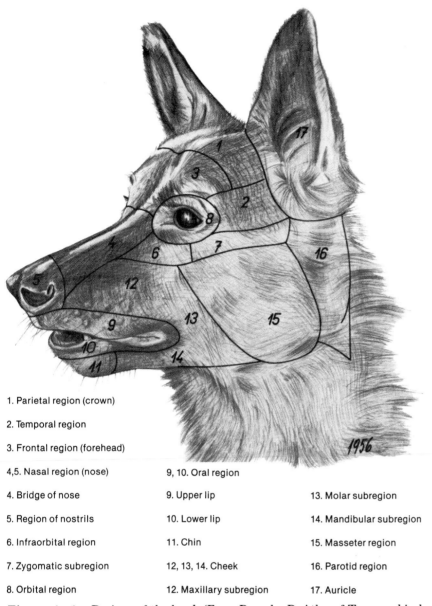

1. Parietal region (crown)

2. Temporal region

3. Frontal region (forehead)

4,5. Nasal region (nose)

4. Bridge of nose

5. Region of nostrils

6. Infraorbital region

7. Zygomatic subregion

8. Orbital region

9, 10. Oral region

9. Upper lip

10. Lower lip

11. Chin

12, 13, 14. Cheek

12. Maxillary subregion

13. Molar subregion

14. Mandibular subregion

15. Masseter region

16. Parotid region

17. Auricle

Figure 4 – 1. Regions of the head. (From Popesko P: Atlas of Topographical Anatomy of the Domestic Animals, 2nd ed. Philadelphia, WB Saunders, 1977.)

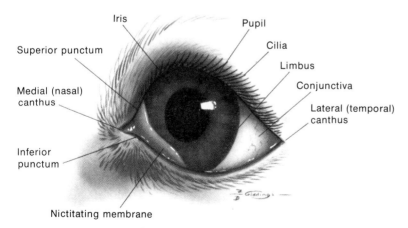

Figure 4 – 2. The eye and periocular structures. (From Slatter DH: Fundamentals of Veterinary Ophthalmology. Philadelphia, WB Saunders, 1981.)

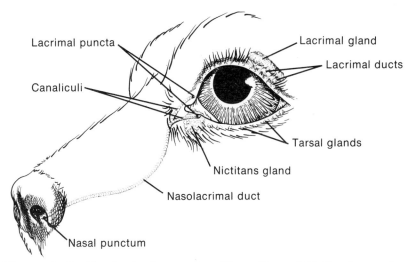

Figure 4–3. Nasolacrimal apparatus. (From Slatter DH: Fundamentals of Veterinary Ophthalmology, p 324. Philadelphia, WB Saunders, 1981.)

The external **ear** is composed of the pinna, the funnel-shaped cartilage that guides sound vibrations to the tympanic membrane, and the horizontal and vertical canals. The shape of the pinna depends on the breed and any cosmetic surgery that has been done to alter it. Figure 4–4 illustrates the anatomy of the external ear. The middle ear or tympanic cavity houses the auditory ossicles, the chordae tympani branch of the facial nerve, muscles, and the auditory tube. The tympanic membrane marks the entrance to the middle ear. The otoscopic view of the tympanic membrane and the middle ear is shown in Figure 4–5. The inner ear is not visible but consists of the membranous labyrinth, a system of fluid-filled sacs and canals, which is housed in the bony labyrinth.

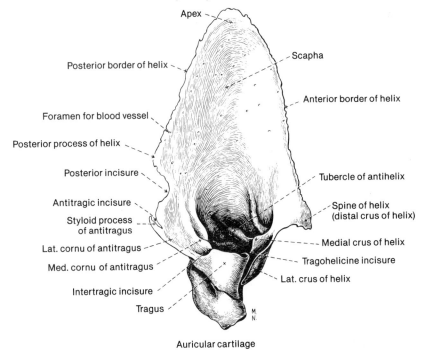

Figure 4–4. Anatomy of the external ear. (Used by permission. From Getty R, Foust HL, Presley ET, Miller ME: Macroscopic anatomy of the ear of the dog. Am J Vet Res 17:364–375, 1956.)

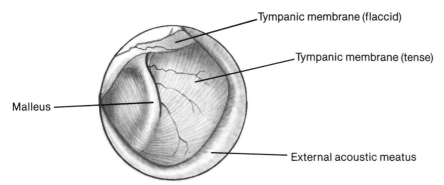

Figure 4-5. View of the normal tympanum of a dog through an otoscope.

The **paranasal sinuses** are air-filled spaces within the skull that are lined with a mucous membrane (Fig. 4-6). The frontal sinuses occupy the dorsal part of the skull between the nasal cavity, the cranium, and the orbits. The frontal sinus of the dog has three compartments: lateral, medial, and rostral frontal sinuses. The maxillary sinus of the dog is located ventral to the orbit at the level of the fourth premolar and first molar.

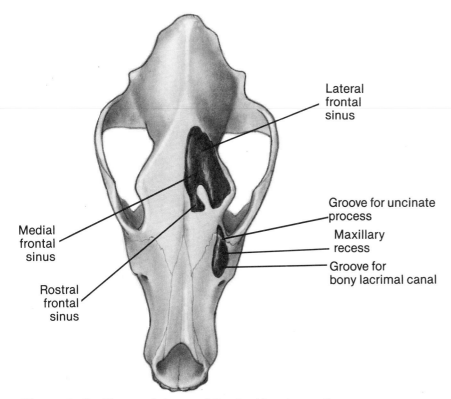

Figure 4-6. Paranasal sinuses of the dog (dorsal aspect).

Three **salivary glands** are of importance in the dog and cat (Fig. 4-7). The most readily palpable is the mandibular salivary gland, which is located ventral and medial to the angle of the mandible below the wing of the atlas. It is oval, well-encapsulated, and firm in texture. The parotid salivary gland is small and triangular in shape, with the apex pointing ventrally. There are two sublingual salivary

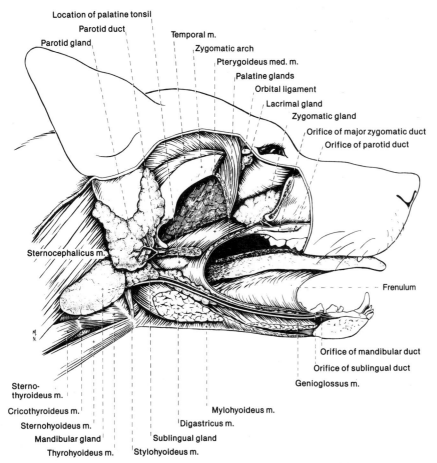

Location of palatine tonsil
Parotid duct
Parotid gland
Temporal m.
Zygomatic arch
Pterygoideus med. m.
Palatine glands
Orbital ligament
Lacrimal gland
Zygomatic gland
Orifice of major zygomatic duct
Orifice of parotid duct
Sternocephalicus m.
Frenulum
Orifice of mandibular duct
Orifice of sublingual duct
Genioglossus m.
Sterno-thyroideus m.
Cricothyroideus m.
Mylohyoideus m.
Sternohyoideus m.
Digastricus m.
Mandibular gland
Sublingual gland
Thyrohyoideus m.
Stylohyoideus m.

Figure 4–7. Location of the salivary glands in the dog. (Used by permission. From Evans HB, Christensen GC: Miller's Anatomy of the Dog, 2nd ed. Philadelphia, WB Saunders, 1979.)

glands, a monostomatic (one duct) and a polystomatic (multiple ducts). The monostomatic gland is located just rostral to the mandibular salivary gland medial to the ramus of the mandible. The polystomatic gland is made up of 6 to 12 lobules under the oral mucosa on each side of the tongue.

The upper and lower **lips** are a mucocutaneous junction and mark the entrance to the oral cavity. The vestibule of the mouth is that space outside the teeth and gums and inside the cheeks and lips. The limits of the oral cavity proper are the hard palate dorsally, the dental arcades laterally and rostrally, and the tongue and mucosa ventrally.

The **teeth** are highly specialized structures in carnivores. The dental formulas of the dog and cat are listed in Table 4–1. The deciduous incisor and canine teeth erupt at about 3 to 4 weeks of age, and the premolar and molar teeth erupt at 5 to 6 weeks of age. Replacement of the incisors, canines, premolars, and molars occurs at 2 to 5 months, 5 to 6 months, 4 to 6 months, and 5 to 7 months, respectively.

Table 4–1
DENTAL FORMULAS OF DOGS AND CATS

	Incisors	Canine	Premolars	Molars
Dog				
Deciduous				
Upper	3	1	3	0
Lower	3	1	3	0
Adult				
Upper	3	1	4	2
Lower	3	1	4	3
Cat				
Deciduous				
Upper	3	1	3	0
Lower	3	1	2	0
Adult				
Upper	3	1	3	1
Lower	3	1	2	1

The **tongue** has an apex, body, and root. The mucous membrane of the tongue is thickened dorsally and is modified to have papillae. The filiform and conical papillae have a mechanical function and are located on the dorsum of the tongue. The vallate, fungiform, and foliate papillae are involved in taste sensation. The fungiform papillae are concentrated on the borders and lateral surfaces of the tongue, the vallate papillae at the root, and the foliate papillae immediately rostral to the palatoglossal arch.

The **pharynx** is composed of three parts: the nasopharynx, which is dorsal to the soft palate; the oropharynx, which is bounded by the root of the tongue, the epiglottis, and the soft palate; and the laryngopharynx, which is that portion of the pharynx immediately rostral to the larynx and caudal to the epiglottis (Fig. 4–8). Within the pharynx are the tonsils. The most prominent is the palatine tonsil, which lies in the tonsillar fossa in the lateral walls of the oropharynx rostral to the palatoglossal fold. The lingual and pharyngeal tonsils and the tonsil of the soft palate are diffuse accumulations of lymphoid tissue in their respective areas of the pharynx.

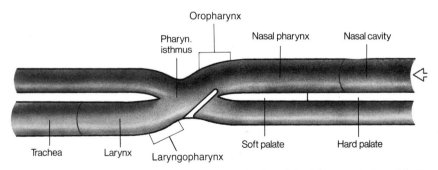

Figure 4–8. Anatomy of the pharynx in the dog. (Used by permission. Modified from Evans HB, Christensen GC: Miller's Anatomy of the Dog, 2nd ed. Philadelphia, WB Saunders, 1979.)

The **larynx** is the cartilaginous structure that forms the entrance to the respiratory system. It is composed of separate cartilage components that vary in their shape between the dog and cat. The anatomy of the larynx is illustrated in Figure 4–9.

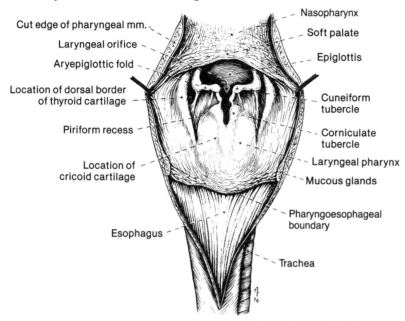

Figure 4–9. Anatomy of the larynx in the dog. (From Evans HB, Christensen GC: Miller's Anatomy of the Dog, 2nd ed. Philadelphia, WB Saunders, 1979.)

The **lymph nodes** of the head and neck of importance are the mandibular, retropharyngeal, and superficial cervical (Fig. 4–10). The mandibular lymph nodes, usually paired, are just rostral to the mandibular salivary gland on either side of the linguofacial vein. They are ovoid and flattened and approximately 1 cm in diameter.

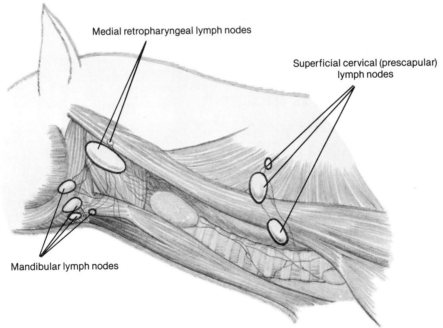

Figure 4–10. Superficial lymph nodes of importance in the head and neck region. (Modified from Evans HB, Christensen GC: Miller's Anatomy of the Dog, 2nd ed. Philadelphia, WB Saunders, 1979.)

The medial retropharyngeal lymph node lies under the wing of the atlas just caudal to the digastric muscle. The lateral retropharyngeal lymph node is inconsistently found along the dorsal border of the mandibular salivary gland. The superficial cervical or prescapular lymph node is present along the anterior border of the supraspinatus covered by the omotransverse and brachiocephalic muscles.

The **trachea** marks the midline of the neck. On either side of the trachea are the muscles that form the jugular groove, which contains the external jugular vein. The sternocephalic muscle forms the medial border and the cleidocephalic muscle forms the lateral border. Deep to the sternocephalic muscle lies the carotid sheath, which contains the common carotid artery, the internal jugular vein, and the vagosympathetic trunk. Dorsally on the neck, the wings of the atlas can be found immediately caudal to the base of the ear. The neck musculature of the dog and cat is heavy dorsally; however, the transverse processes of the cervical vertebrae are readily palpable.

Observation

As the examination begins, note the symmetry and posture of the head. Does the animal have a head tilt? Does the animal seem to be reluctant to move the head? Are there any swellings of the head or face? Are the lips symmetric? Is the nose drawn to one side?

A head tilt is indicative of vestibular disease.

Reluctance to move the head may indicate neck pain, as in the case of cervical disc disease or meningitis.

Facial nerve paralysis results in a drooping of the lip on the affected side (Fig. 4–11). Contracture of the facial muscles occurs after prolonged denervation.

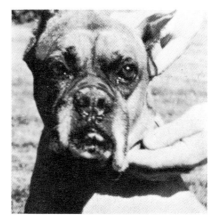

Figure 4–11. Facial nerve paralysis. Note the drooped lip on the left side of the face. (Used by permission. From Oliver JE Jr, Hoerlein BF, Mayhew IG: Veterinary Neurology. Philadelphia, WB Saunders, 1984.)

Note the skin and hair over the head and neck. Are there any areas of alopecia? Are discolorations, rashes, or masses present on the skin? The inner surface of the pinna is a good place to look for abnormalities in color or evidence of hemorrhage. Observe the area of the jugular groove for a visible pulse.

Pale pinnae are indicative of anemia or poor peripheral circulation. A yellow color is seen with jaundice (Fig. 4–12).

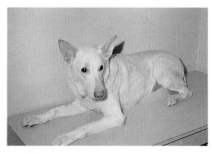

Figure 4–12. Discoloration of the pinna is indicative of icterus.

The presence of a jugular pulse indicates right heart failure or other obstruction to venous return.

The nose should be examined for symmetry, texture, and color. The presence of any discharge and its character should be noted. The movement of air from each nostril can be estimated by placing a glass slide or mirror in front of one nostril and watching the slide for fogging (Fig. 4–13). The area of fogging should be the same for each nostril.

Nasal discharge may result from infectious causes, including canine tooth root abscess, neoplasia, and foreign body penetration.

Decreased movement of air from one nostril may be a result of obstruction of the nasal passage with exudate, a neoplasm, or a foreign object. In brachycephalic dogs, the nostril openings may be too small for easy movement of air during inspiration, a condition known as stenotic nares.

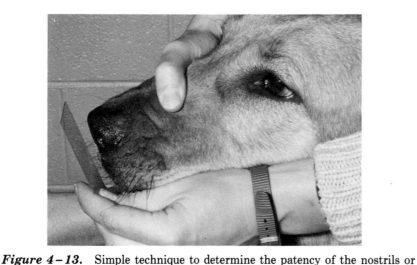

Figure 4–13. Simple technique to determine the patency of the nostrils or nasal passages is shown. A glass slide is placed in front of the nose and the area of fogging is compared for each side.

Examination of the eyes and periocular structures follows. First, look at the eyes from in front of the animal. Are both eyes looking in the same direction? Are the palpebral fissures symmetric? Is there any nystagmus present at rest? Looking at the animal from above or the side, are both eyes seated well within the orbit? Examine the

Strabismus indicates dysfunction of the extraocular muscles innervated by cranial nerves III, IV, or VI (Fig. 4–14).

edges of the eyelids for eyelash placement. Are there lashes directed toward the eye (Fig. 4–15)? Are there any reddened or swollen areas along the lid margins? Do the lid margins contact the cornea? Is the conjunctiva red and inflamed? Note the presence of ocular discharge. The corneas should be examined for opacities and smoothness. The visible portion of the lens should be transparent. A transilluminator or penlight can be used to elicit the direct and consensual pupillary light responses as well as the tapetal reflex. (The pupillary light response is covered in detail in Chapter 11.) In addition, the light can demonstrate small corneal defects. The iris may be one of a variety of colors, but the apertures should be symmetric. Note any swelling, localized or generalized, of the iris.

Text continued on page 37

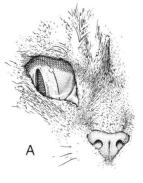

A

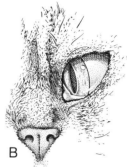

B

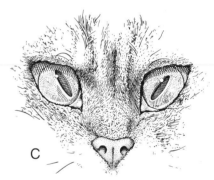

C

Figure 4–14. Strabismus is indicated when the eyes are not aligned in the same direction. Directions of strabismus are shown following paralysis of the *(A)* oculomotor, *(B)* abducens, and *(C)* trochlear neurons. (Used by permission. From de Lahunta A: Veterinary Neuroanatomy and Clinical Neurology. Philadelphia, WB Saunders, 1977.)

Nystagmus can be present with vestibular or cerebellar disease.

An eye that protrudes may be either enlarged (buphthalmic) or not well seated in the socket (exophthalmic). An eye that appears sunken may be small (microphthalmic) or enophthalmic.

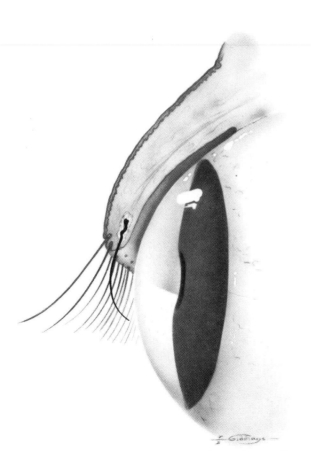

Figure 4–15. Distichia are eyelashes that are directed inward toward the cornea. (Used by permission. From Slatter DH: Fundamentals of Veterinary Ophthalmology, p 210. Philadelphia, WB Saunders, 1981.)

Distichia are eyelashes that are directed inward toward the cornea, which can result in corneal irritation or ulceration.

Entropion and ectropion are common lid abnormalities in dogs, which result in corneal trauma (Figs. 4–16 and 4–17).

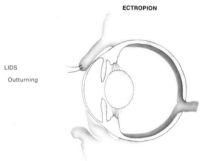

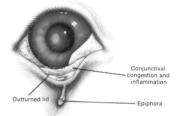

Figure 4–16. Failure of the lower lid to contact the cornea due to redundant tissue is termed ectropion. (Used by permission. From Slatter DH: Fundamentals of Veterinary Ophthalmology, p 227. Philadelphia, WB Saunders, 1981.)

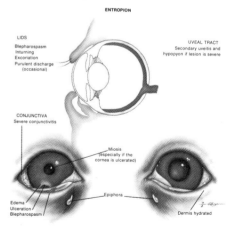

Figure 4–17. Inward rolling of the upper and/or lower eyelids such that the hair or eyelashes are against the cornea is entropion. (Used by permission. From Slatter DH: Fundamentals of Veterinary Ophthalmology, p 225. Philadelphia, WB Saunders, 1981.)

Table 4–2 illustrates examples of common ocular disorders detected on physical examination. Conjunctivitis results in reddened, inflamed conjunctiva. Often a discharge is present but the eye itself is unaffected. Uveitis may also result in conjunctival reddening, but in this case the pupil is miotic and there is evidence of pain in the affected eye (photophobia, blepharospasm).

Table 4–2
COMMON OCULAR ABNORMALITIES DETECTED ON A PHYSICAL EXAMINATION

Disorder	Example
Eyelids	
Tarsal gland adenoma Benign tumor of the eyelid	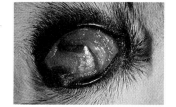
Distichiasis Abnormal eyelash position	
Prolapse of the glans nictitans Also referred to as cherry eye	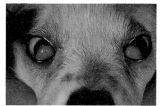
Everted cartilage of the glans nictitans The cartilage of the third eyelid can be seen curled on itself *(arrows).*	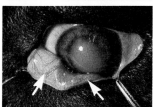
Conjunctiva	
Foreign body A grass awn is easily seen in the conjunctival sac.	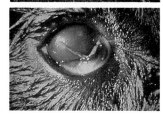

Table continued on the following page

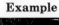

Table 4–2 *continued*

Disorder	**Example**
Conjunctivitis (bacterial) A bacterial infection of the conjunctiva causing discharge, redness, and pain	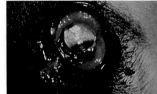
Keratoconjunctivitis sicca The lack of tear production causes corneal and conjunctival irritation.	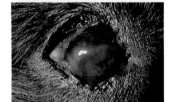
Subconjunctival hemorrhage	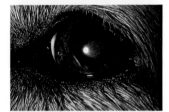
Cornea **Corneal ulcer** A disruption in the corneal epithelium	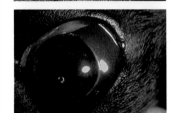
Corneal dystrophy Cholesterol deposits in the corneal stroma	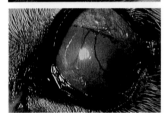
German Shepherd pannus Vascular and pigmentary migration across the cornea	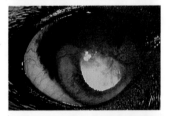
Eosinophilic keratitis A condition in cats in which eosinophils infiltrate the cornea	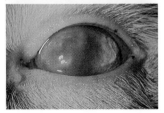

Table 4–2 *continued*

Disorder	Example
Anterior chamber	
Hemorrhage	
Hypopyon Pus in the anterior chamber	
Lens luxation The lens is displaced into the anterior chamber.	
Anterior uveitis An inflammatory condition of the eye, which is characterized by pain, miosis, redness, and decreased intraocular pressure	
Acute glaucoma Increased intraocular pressure associated with mydriasis, pain, and redness	
Chronic glaucoma Chronic increased intraocular pressure results in enlargement of the eye (buphthalmia) and blindness.	
Iris Atrophy Degenerative change in the iris causing holes to form	

Table continued on the following page

Table 4–2 *continued*

Disorder	Example
Iris prolapse through a corneal ulcer Severe ulceration of the cornea associated with rupture of Descemet's membrane and loss of fluid from the anterior chamber (*arrow* points to the iris)	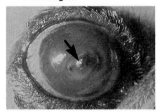

Photographs courtesy of Dr. Glenn Severin, Colorado State University, College of Veterinary Medicine and Biomedical Sciences.

White opacities on the cornea can be a result of corneal edema, corneal scars, or corneal dystrophies. Chronic superficial pigmentary keratitis, or pannus, causes a dark brown or black discoloration of the cornea.

Cataracts prohibit the visualization of the tapetal reflex because the lens is opaque. Nuclear sclerosis, a common aging phenomenon in the lens, does not result in the loss of the tapetal reflex.

Anisocoria is asymmetry in pupil size (Fig. 4–18). Table 4–3 lists the causes of anisocoria. Iris atrophy results in a large pupil with irregular edges and may be confused with anisocoria if each pupil is affected to a variable degree.

Table 4–3
CAUSES OF ANISOCORIA

Cause	Pupil Size (Affected Eye)	Pupillary Light Response* DIRECT	INDIRECT	Dark Response
Anterior uveitis	Small	Already small	Normal	Sluggish
Horner's syndrome	Medium	Normal	Normal	None
Posterior synechia	Small	No response	Normal	None
Primary glaucoma	Large	No response	Normal if retina intact; no response if retina damaged	Already dilated
Progressive retinal atrophy	Large	No response	No response	Already dilated
Oculomotor nerve disease	Large	No response	Normal	Already dilated
Optic nerve	Large	No response	No response	Already dilated

* Assume a unilateral lesion: direct = light shining in affected eye, response in that eye; indirect = light shining in affected eye, response in the other eye.

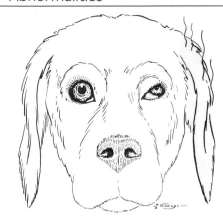

1. Ptosis
2. Miosis
3. Prominent membrana nictitans
4. Enophthalmos
5. Warm, pink ear
6. Sweating on face and neck
   in horses

Figure 4–18. Clinical signs of Horner's syndrome. Note the unequal size of the pupillary apertures. (Used by permission. From Slatter DH: Fundamentals of Veterinary Ophthalmology, p 608. Philadelphia, WB Saunders, 1981.)

An ophthalmoscope can be used to examine the retina after proper pupil dilation. The room should be dimly lit for this procedure. Set the ophthalmoscope at 0 diopters initially. Place the ophthalmoscope in front of your eye, resting on the brow (Fig. 4–19). Slowly advance toward the animal until the scope is at the level of the animal's nose. Use your right eye and right hand to look at the patient's right eye and your left eye and left hand to look at the patient's left eye. This allows for a more mobile examination. Try to keep both eyes open and relaxed. Survey the retina in a systematic manner, paying close attention to the vessels and optic disc. Usually in small animals, a negative (red) 3-diopter setting is required to bring the retina into sharp focus. To look at the lens and vitreous, a positive (black) 10-diopter setting is necessary.

Table 4–4 gives examples of ocular abnormalities detected with an ophthalmoscope.

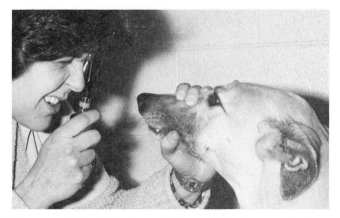

Figure 4–19. Technique of direct ophthalmoscopy is shown.

Table 4-4
**OCULAR ABNORMALITIES OBSERVED WITH
AN OPHTHALMOSCOPE**

Type	Cause
Light-absorbing Hyporeflective	Congenital
	Absence of a tapetum
	Pigment over tapetum
	Retinal dysplasia
	Acquired
	Retinitis
	Hemorrhage
	Retinal detachment
	Lens luxation
Light-reflecting Hyper-reflective	Congenital
	Progressive retinal degeneration
	Retinal dysplasia
	Acquired
	Inactive retinitis
	Retinal detachment
	Central retinal degeneration
Miscellaneous	Congenital
	Collie eye anomaly
	Acquired
	Optic neuritis

The response, or lack thereof, to noises should be noted. If the ability of the animal to hear is questionable, clapping behind the animal's head in such a way that it cannot see the motion should elicit a startle response if the hearing is all right. The carriage of the ears should be symmetric and the movement of the ears to various stimuli lively. Is the external ear canal reddened or ulcerated? Is there exudate within the canal? Does the animal shake its head or scratch its ears frequently during the examination?

One ear may be carried lower than the other if it is inflamed or if an aural hematoma is present (Fig. 4-20). Aural hematomas are usually secondary to otitis externa or foreign bodies within the ear.

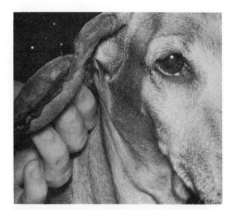

Figure 4-20. Aural hematoma is a common cause of swelling of the pinna and asymmetric ear carriage. (Courtesy of Dr. Howard Seim, Colorado State University.)

Otitis externa is a common ear problem in certain breeds of dogs, such as cocker spaniels, poodles, and golden retrievers. It arises from a variety of causes and results in a painful, inflamed ear with variable quantities of exudate within the canal. A brown, odorous exudate is typical of yeast infections. A bacterial otitis may give rise to a yellowish discharge. Head shaking is indicative of otitis externa or aural foreign body.

At this point, an otoscopic examination can be performed to better view the vertical and horizontal canals and the tympanic membrane. The animal should be restrained by placing one arm around the neck so that the inner surface of the elbow is under the animal's mandible. Grasp the pinna with the thumb and forefinger of the left hand and gently pull it dorsally. The remaining fingers of that hand can be used as a brace against the animal's head so that sudden movements are less likely to result in damage to the ear. The cone of the otoscope is then placed in the vertical canal and, as you examine the canal, advance around the angle into the horizontal canal (Fig. 4–21). Normal cerumen is usually white or light tan in color. The canal should be free of debris and exudate. The skin of the canal should be pale pink without evidence of ulceration, scaling, or masses. The normal tympanic membrane is translucent and somewhat concave (see Fig. 4–5 and Table 4–5). The attachment of the manubrium of the malleus to the membrane is visible as a white streak running dorsocaudally.

Plant awns are common foreign objects within the ear canal.

Chronic otitis externa can result in proliferation of polypoid masses within the ear canal. In addition, the ear canal usually is inflamed and contains exudate.

Table 4–5 illustrates abnormalities that may be observed within the ear canal.

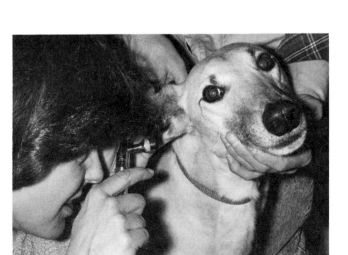

Figure 4–21. Otoscopic examination.

Table 4-5
COMMON ABNORMALITIES OF THE EXTERNAL EAR IDENTIFIED BY OTOSCOPIC EXAMINATION

Disorder	Example
Normal typanic membrane	
Otodectes canis (ear mites)	
Rupture of tympanic membrane	
Foreign body (foxtail)	
Inflammatory polyps	

Photographs courtesy of Dr. Patrick McKeever, University of Minnesota, College of Veterinary Medicine.

Examine the lips for color, lumps, ulcers, or cracking. The buccal and gingival mucosa should be inspected for color, hemorrhages, ulcers, and masses. The condition of the teeth should also be noted, paying special attention to the presence or absence of teeth, tartar build-up, looseness of teeth, and damage to teeth. Inspect the color

Petechial hemorrhages are indicative of thrombocytopenia or other coagulopathy (Fig. 4-22). Gingivitis varies in severity and is evidenced by red discoloration of

and form of the hard and soft palates. Note the symmetry, color, and texture of the tongue. Using the index finger to depress the body of the tongue, examine the pharynx for abnormalities in color, texture, and mucosal lining. The palatine tonsils are normally within the fossae and not readily visible. A gag reflex should be elicited by stimulating the pharynx with your finger.

the gingiva near the teeth (Fig. 4-23). Ulceration and proliferation of gingival tissue occur as the disease progresses.

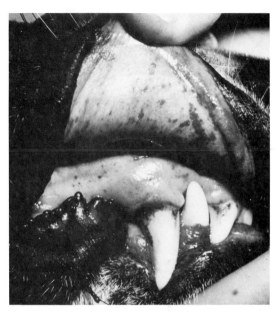

Figure 4-22. Petechial hemorrhages on the oral mucosa of a dog with immune-mediated thrombocytopenia.

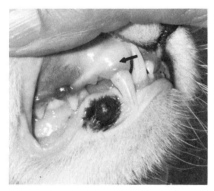

Figure 4-23. Line of discoloration *(arrow)* along the gingiva near the teeth is indicative of mild gingivitis.

Neoplastic masses involving the palate result in loss of symmetry and often ulceration of the mucosa.

Enlarged tonsils are easily seen protruding from the fossae. Local inflammation or systemic illness such as lymphosarcoma may result in enlargement of the tonsils.

Palpation

Palpate the face and skull for defects in symmetry and bony structure. Crepitus may indicate fractures of the bones or subcutaneous emphysema. Is pain evident on palpation? The texture and size of the mandibular and superficial cervical lymph nodes should be noted. Palpate along the trachea, between the laryngeal cartilages and the thoracic inlet, for the thyroid glands. Gentle squeezing of the trachea may elicit a cough. Palpate the base of the ear and the pinna and note any pain or swelling. Are there any parasites present around the head and neck? With the patient's eyelids closed, compare the ocular pressure of both eyes by gently pressing on the eyes simultaneously.

Nasal tumors may cause erosion of the nasal bone over the dorsum of the face. This can be palpated as a soft depression in the affected area.

Normal thyroid glands are usually nonpalpable.

Easily elicited coughs are indicative of tracheal inflammation. Causes may include infectious tracheobronchitis and tracheal collapse.

Pain along the base of the ear may indicate otitis externa.

A softer than normal eye indicates uveitis. Glaucoma results in increased intraocular pressure.

Auscultation

Auscultate the trachea and laryngeal areas.

A high-pitched wheeze on inspiration (stridor) indicates an upper airway obstruction such as laryngeal paralysis.

Percussion

Percuss the area of the frontal sinus.

Fluid within the sinuses results in a dulling of the sound transmission.

DIFFERENCES IN THE CAT

Be sure to carefully examine under the cat's tongue. This can be done by placing the thumb of one hand in the intermandibular space and pressing upward, followed by probing the area under the tongue with the index finger of the same hand (Fig. 4–24).

By carefully examining under the tongue, a string foreign body may be visualized as it wraps around the base of the tongue. Ulceration and mucosal proliferation are seen with lymphocytic-plasmacytic stomatitis (Fig. 4–25) (see following page).

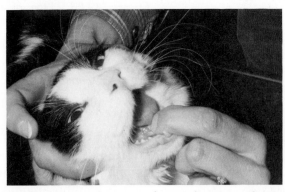

Figure 4–24. To examine the area under a cat's tongue, place a thumb in the intermandibular space and, while applying gentle upward pressure, lift the tongue with the index finger.

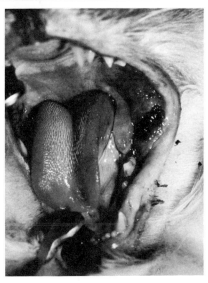

The paraepiglottic tonsil is found only in the cat and is located on the base of the epiglottis.

Note that cats have elliptic pupils.

Thyroid adenomas are common in older cats and can be palpated anywhere between the larynx and the thoracic inlet (Fig. 4–26).

Figure 4–25. Stomatitis is indicated by the red, roughened, and ulcerated oral mucosa.

Purring can often be a hindrance to auscultation in the cat. There are several tricks to use to attempt to stop the purring. Holding the cat near the edge of the table may be enough in some cats. More drastic measures include flicking the cat's nose with a finger or holding the cat near a sink with the water running slowly. Always explain to the client what you are doing.

The frontal sinuses in the cat are very small and undivided. There is no maxillary sinus of importance in the cat.

The dental formula in the cat is different from that in the dog, as previously mentioned. The cat's tongue is especially cornified and rough for grooming purposes.

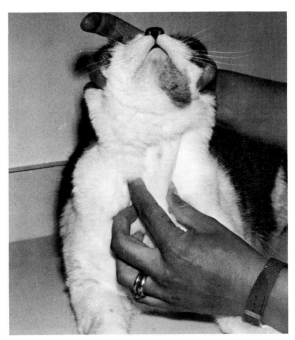

Figure 4–26. Palpation for the thyroid glands in the cat.

RECOMMENDED READING

1. Bates B: A Guide to Physical Diagnosis and History Taking, 4th ed. Philadelphia, JB Lippincott, 1987.
2. Bistner S, Shaw D: Examination of the eye. Vet Clin North Am, 11(3):595–622, 1981.
3. Kirk RW, Bistner SI: Handbook of Veterinary Procedures and Emergency Treatment, 3rd ed. Philadelphia, WB Saunders, 1981.
4. Miller ME, Christensen GC, Evans HE: Anatomy of the Dog. Philadelphia, WB Saunders, 1964.
5. Muller GH, Kirk RW, Scott DW: Small Animal Dermatology, 3rd ed. Philadelphia, WB Saunders, 1983.
6. Severin GA: Veterinary Ophthalmology class notes. Colorado State University, Ft. Collins, CO, 1976.
7. Slatter DH: Fundamentals of Veterinary Ophthalmology. Philadelphia, WB Saunders, 1981.
8. Wyman M: Manual of Small Animal Ophthalmology. New York, Churchill Livingstone, 1986.

Respiratory System

APPLIED ANATOMY

Review the anatomy of the chest wall (Fig. 5–1). To localize and describe an abnormality, ribs and interspaces must be counted accurately. In the dog and cat, this can be done by counting backwards from the thirteenth rib or by locating the fifth rib, which is usually at the level of the point of the olecranon if the limb is in the normal standing position. The cartilages of the first nine ribs articulate directly with the sternum. The cartilages of ribs ten, eleven, and twelve form the costal arch, and rib thirteen floats freely. The tip of the thirteenth rib can usually be felt caudodorsolaterally on the thorax. Another helpful landmark is the caudal border of the scapula, which is at the level of the fifth to sixth rib.

The thoracic cavity occupies only the cranial aspect of the bony thorax; therefore, the thoracic cavity is smaller than the bony thorax. It changes size with respiration. The line of pleural reflection approximates a line drawn from just below the costochondral junction of the eighth rib through the costochondral junction of the eleventh rib to the dorsal part of the thirteenth rib. This line marks the caudoventral extent of the costodiaphragmatic recess. Incisions caudal to this line enter the abdomen. It is helpful to know the approximate location of the lungs (Fig. 5–2). The left lung is divided into cranial and caudal lobes. The cranial lobe has cranial and caudal parts. The right lung is divided into cranial, middle, caudal, and accessory lobes. The cardiac notch, between the right cranial and middle lung lobes, is at the level of the fourth and fifth interspaces. A small portion of each lung extends anterior to the first rib. The cranial lobe of the right lung ends at the level of the fourth to sixth rib. The caudal lobe begins at the level of the sixth rib. On the left, the cranial lobe ends at about the fifth interspace and the caudal

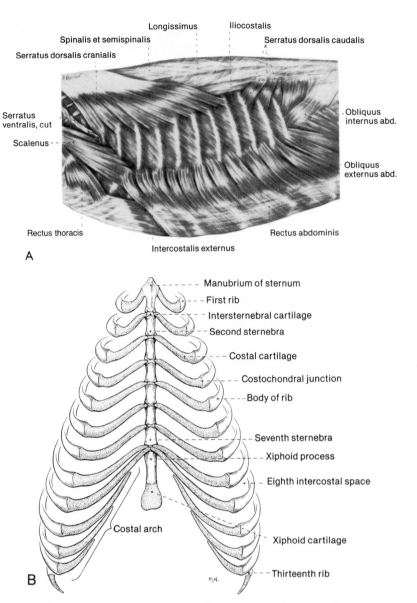

Longissimus
Iliocostalis
Spinalis et semispinalis
Serratus dorsalis caudalis
Serratus dorsalis cranialis

Serratus
ventralis, cut
Obliquus
internus abd.

Scalenus
Obliquus
externus abd.

Rectus thoracis
Rectus abdominis

Intercostalis externus

A

Manubrium of sternum

First rib

Intersternebral cartilage

Second sternebra

Costal cartilage

Costochondral junction

Body of rib

Seventh sternebra

Xiphoid process

Eighth intercostal space

Costal arch

Xiphoid cartilage

Thirteenth rib

B

Figure 5 – 1. Anatomy of the thoracic wall: *A,* superficial muscles (lateral aspect). *B,* Ribs and sternum (ventral aspect). (Used by permission. From Evans HB, Christensen GC: Miller's Anatomy of the Dog, 2nd ed. Philadelphia, WB Saunders, 1979.)

lobe begins there. The diaphragm attaches to the thirteenth rib dorsocaudally and slopes anteroventrally to attach onto the eighth, ninth, and tenth ribs. It bells forward to the level of the sixth rib. In the normal animal, the diaphragm moves one to one and one-half spaces forward and back during respiration. The bifurcation of the trachea into the mainstem bronchi is in the centrodorsal thorax at the level of the fourth interspace.

The pleural space in the normal living animal is only a potential space. It lies between the visceral and parietal pleura and is normally occupied by a small amount of pleural fluid.

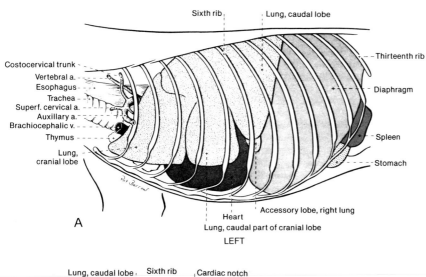

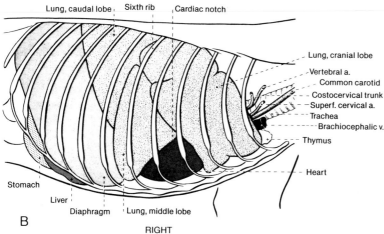

Figure 5–2. Location of the lungs within the bony thorax. *A,* Left superficial lateral view. *B,* Right superficial lateral view. (Used by permission. From Evans HB, Christensen GC: Miller's Anatomy of the Dog, 2nd ed. Philadelphia, WB Saunders, 1979.)

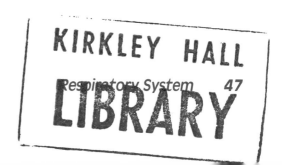

Observation

Observe the respiratory pattern, noting the rate, depth, rhythm, and effort. The normal breathing of an animal at rest is quiet and regular at a rate of 10 to 30 per minute. See Table 5–1 for an explanation of abnormal respiratory patterns. Note the shape of the chest and its movements. What is the animal's posture? Does the animal look comfortable? Is the animal open-mouth breathing? Note the color of the mucous membranes. Is there any coughing or sneezing? Does the animal have a nasal discharge? If so, what is the character of the discharge?

An animal that has increased respiratory efforts may have a barrel-shaped chest. Animals with severe dyspnea often stand with elbows abducted. Extension of the head and neck are also characteristic of severe dyspnea. A red, frothy nasal discharge is indicative of pulmonary hemorrhage, whereas a pale pink froth is usually associated with pulmonary edema. A purulent nasal discharge can be seen with bacterial bronchopneumonia or upper respiratory infections (Fig. 5–3).

Table 5–1
ABNORMAL RESPIRATORY PATTERNS

Character	Associated Conditions
Rapid, shallow (tachypnea)	Restrictive pattern seen with thoracic effusions, pneumothorax, diaphragmatic hernia
Rapid, deep (hyperpnea)	Acidosis, fever, exercise, excitement
Slow, normal depth (bradypnea)	Respiratory depression, coma, increased intracranial pressure
Slow, deep	Obtructive pattern seen with laryngeal paralysis, tracheal collapse/compression

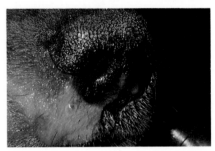

Figure 5–3. Purulent nasal discharge.

Palpation

Palpate the larynx, trachea, and thorax. Is the thorax symmetric? Are there any masses or swellings? Note any rib abnormalities. Are there any tender areas? Further assess the respiratory pattern by palpation. Is there symmetry to the movements of the chest? Are vibrations or crepitant areas felt?

Chondrosarcomas or other neoplasms of the ribs often result in a firm, nonpainful swelling of the rib. Rib fractures are painful and crepitant on palpation.

Auscultation

With the diaphragm portion of the stethoscope, listen to the breath sounds from the larynx down to the thorax. Nine areas on each side of the thorax are usually auscultated depending on the size of the animal (Fig. 5–4). To maximize the quality of information gained by this technique, it is wise to have a comfortable, well-fit stethoscope and to use it consistently. The room should be as quiet as possible even if you have to politely ask the client to refrain from talking during this time. Consciously block out cardiac sounds for this part of the examination. Extraneous noises may interfere with auscultation. These arise from muscular trembling, hair rubbing against the stethoscope, and background music or noise. In the normal animal, breath sounds can be heard throughout inspiration and during the first third of expiration. Refer to Table 5–2 for a review of abnormal or adventitious breath sounds. The tidal volume

Palpable vibrations within the chest are associated with exudation within the respiratory tract.

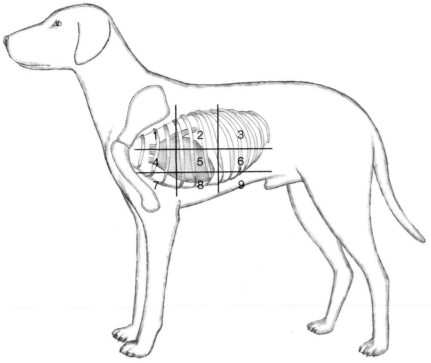

Figure 5–4. Nine areas of thoracic auscultation.

Table 5–2 ABNORMAL RESPIRATORY SOUNDS		
Type	**Description**	**Associated Conditions**
Breath sounds	Louder than normal, pronounced on inspiration	Increased ventilation, consolidation, lung mass, obstructive airway disease
Breath sounds	Softer than normal	Hyperinflation, emphysema, pneumothorax, thoracic effusion, diaphragmatic hernia
Adventitious sounds Crackles	Nonmuscial, short bursts of noise	
	Late inspiration	Pulmonary edema, pneumonia, neoplasia
	Early inspiration/ early expiration	Obstructive diseases, bronchopneumonia, tracheobronchial fluid
Wheezes	Continuous, musical noises	
	Inspiration	Extrathoracic airway obstruction (laryngeal paralysis, collapsing extrathoracic trachea, foreign body, neoplasia)
	Expiration	Intrathoracic airway obstruction (collapsing intrathoracic trachea, chronic obstructive pulmonary disease, foreign body, neoplasia)

must be near maximal for optimal auscultation. Little, if any, parenchyma is assessed if the animal is breathing shallowly or panting. To stimulate deep breaths, try to hold the mouth closed and pinch the nares for a short period of time, then release the nares and listen as the animal takes a breath. Other methods to stimulate a deep breath include exercising the animal lightly or inducing a cough by palpating the trachea.

Listen and compare the patient's breath sounds to the lung sounds of normal animals. Also compare the right side to the left and inspiration to expiration. If an abnormal sound is heard or if an area of no sound is heard, move the stethoscope around to localize the source. The timing of the abnormal sound is also important. Is it early or late in inspiration or expiration?

Abnormal or adventitious sounds may arise from the upper or lower respiratory tract. To aid in the localization of a disease process, refer to Table 5–3.

Late inspiratory crackles are heard with pulmonary edema, fibrosis, pneumonia, and neoplastic diseases of the chest wall, pleura, or lung. Early inspiratory crackles may be heard with obstructive disease, bronchopneumonia, or tracheobronchial fluid accumulation.

Table 5–3
LOCALIZATION OF RESPIRATORY DISEASE

	Upper Respiratory Tract	Lower Respiratory Tract
Sneeze	+	–
Cough	+	+
Nasal discharge	+	+/–
Facial swelling	+/–	–
Stertor	+	–
Voice change	+	–
Inspiratory dyspnea	+	+/–
Expiratory dyspnea	–	+
Hyperpnea	–	+
Abnormal lung sounds	–	+
Restrictive respirations	–	+

Percussion

Percussion of the chest wall produces vibrations that are audible. It aids in determining the consistency of the underlying structures. Because the thoracic wall is elastic and overlies air-filled lungs, it vibrates like the head of a drum when struck. In areas where the body wall covers solid structures (liver, heart), it does not vibrate. The sound waves move through the air in the thorax to the thoracic wall until they meet a solid organ or area. The normal sound of the thorax when percussed is a dull or flat sound compared to the tympanitic sound of an air-filled viscus.

To perform percussion, the middle finger of one hand is placed firmly on the intercostal space and is tapped with the middle finger of the other hand between the distal interphalangeal joint and the fingernail (Fig. 5–5). Percuss over the lung fields in a systematic manner. The interpretation of sounds is illustrated in Table 5–4. Identify and localize any area of abnormal sound. Note any change in position of the line of pleural reflection.

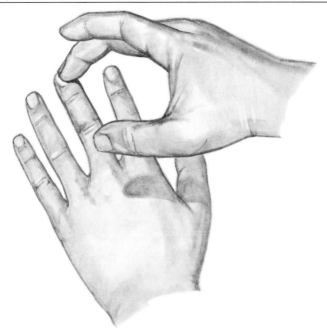

Figure 5-5. Technique of percussion is illustrated.

Table 5-5 summarizes the effects of specific diseases on percussion and auscultation.

Table 5-4
CHARACTERISTIC SOUNDS BY PERCUSSION

Type of Sound	Pitch	Intensity	Duration	Location
Resonant	Low	Loud	Long	Normal lung
Tympanitic	High	Loud	Medium	Gas-filled viscus
Hyper-resonant	Low	Very loud	Long	Pneumothorax, emphysema
Dull	Medium	Soft	Medium	Pleural effusion, neoplasia

Table 5-5
PHYSICAL SIGNS ASSOCIATED WITH COMMON RESPIRATORY TRACT CONDITIONS

Condition	Percussion	Breath Sounds	Adventitious Sounds
Normal	Resonant	Bronchial, bronchovesicular, vesicular	None
Left heart failure	Resonant	Normal	Crackles at lung bases
Pleural fluid	Dull	Decreased or absent ventrally	None (unless underlying lung disease)
Pneumonia	Dull	Bronchial only	Crackles
Bronchitis	Resonant	Prolonged expiration	Crackles, wheezes
Emphysema	Hyper-resonant	Decreased	None
Pneumothorax	Hyper-resonant	Decreased or absent dorsally	None
Atelectasis	Dull	Decreased	None

DIFFERENCES IN THE CAT

Feline respiratory sounds are normally very quiet; thus, if they are readily heard, be suspicious of airway disease. The thorax of the cat is markedly compressible. Gentle but firm pressure between the thumb and fingers allows the anterior chest to be squeezed until the opposite walls touch each other (Fig. 5–6). If this cannot be done, a mass lesion may be present in the anterior mediastinum. Lastly, as already mentioned, purring can be a significant hindrance to auscultation and percussion. The methods previously described can be utilized to inhibit the cat from purring.

Feline asthma is a significant cause of respiratory disease in the cat and can result in increased lung sounds and inspiratory wheezes.

Thymic lymphosarcoma characteristically reduces the compressibility of a cat's chest.

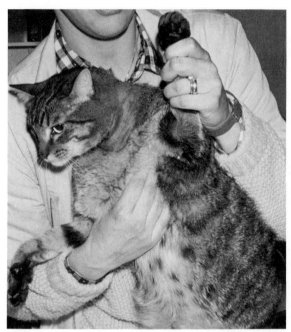

Figure 5–6. The remarkable compressibility of the cat's chest is felt by gently squeezing the anterior thoracic wall between the thumb and four fingers.

RECOMMENDED READING

1. Habel RE: Applied Veterinary Anatomy, 2nd ed. Ithaca, NY, RE Habel, 1981.
2. Kotlikoff MI, Gillespie JR: Lung sounds in veterinary medicine, Part II. Deriving clinical information from lung sounds. Comp Cont Ed 6(5):462–468, 1984.
3. Evans HB, Christensen GC: Miller's Anatomy of the Dog, 2nd ed. Philadelphia, WB Saunders, 1979.
4. Ogburn P, Bistner SI: Examination of the respiratory system. Vet Clin North Am 11(3):623, 1981.

Cardiovascular System

ELLEN M. POFFENBARGER

APPLIED ANATOMY

The heart in the dog is located between the third rib and the sixth interspace (Fig. 6–1). The left ventricle occupies most of the left side of the heart, but because of the way in which the heart is positioned in the thoracic cavity, the anterior part of the right ventricle, the left atrium, and the pulmonary trunk are also on this side. On the right side, the right ventricle occupies the majority of the area, with a small portion of left ventricle caudoventrally and right atrium dorsally (Fig. 6–2). The major vessels of the cardiovascular system within the thorax are the aorta, the pulmonary arteries, and the cranial and caudal venae cavae, which are depicted in Figure 6–1.

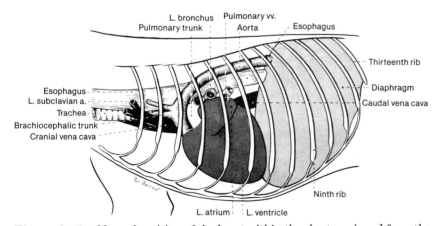

Figure 6–1. Normal position of the heart within the chest as viewed from the left. The major blood vessels within the chest are also visible. (Used by permission. From Evans HB, de Lahunta A: Miller's Guide to the Dissection of the Dog. Philadelphia, WB Saunders, 1971.)

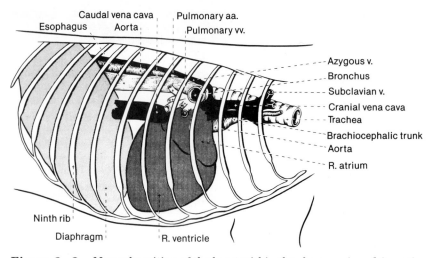

Figure 6–2. *Normal position of the heart within the chest as viewed from the right. (Used by permission. From Evans HB, Christensen GC: Miller's Anatomy of the Dog, 2nd ed. Philadelphia, WB Saunders, 1979.)*

The projection of sound from the various heart valves is shown in Figure 6–3. The point of maximal intensity (that place on the thoracic wall where the loudest sound can be heard) for each valve may not exactly correspond to the anatomic location of the valve.

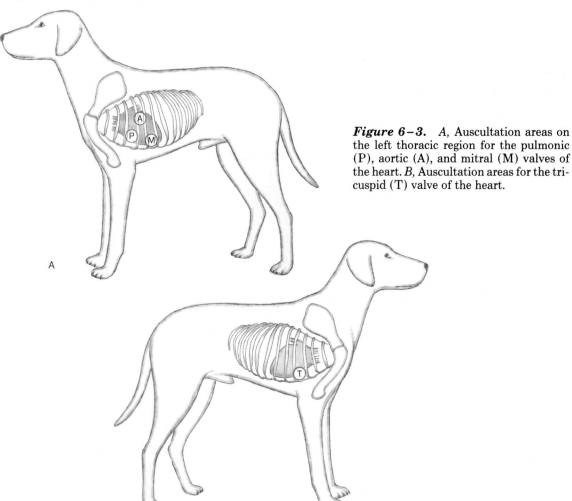

Figure 6–3. *A, Auscultation areas on the left thoracic region for the pulmonic (P), aortic (A), and mitral (M) valves of the heart. B, Auscultation areas for the tricuspid (T) valve of the heart.*

Figure 6–4 depicts the normal heart sounds. The *first heart sound* is generated by the closing of the atrioventricular valves. These are the mitral and tricuspid valves. The point of maximal intensity for the mitral valve is at the level of the fourth to sixth intercostal space just to the left of the sternal border. This area is often referred to as the apex beat or the point on the thorax where the heartbeat can be felt (Fig. 6–5). On the right side of the chest, between the third and fifth interspaces at the level of the costochondral junction, is the point of maximal intensity for the tricuspid valve.

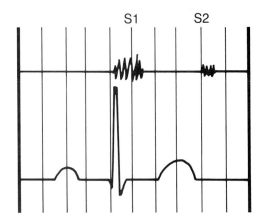

Figure 6–4. Normal heart sounds. The first heart sound (S1) is associated with the closing of the mitral and tricuspid valves. The second heart sound (S2) is associated with the closing of the pulmonic and aortic valves.

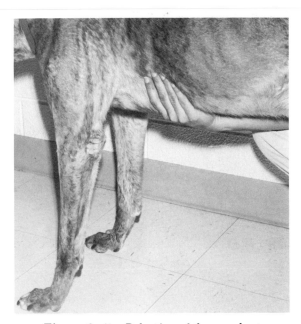

Figure 6–5. Palpation of the apex beat.

The *second heart sound* is generated by the closing of pulmonic and aortic valves. The aortic valve can be heard best on the left side of the thorax in the fourth interspace at the level of the shoulder joint. The best place to auscultate the pulmonic valve is on the left side of the thorax in the second to fourth interspace just above the sternal border.

In the assessment of the cardiovascular system, other vessels of importance include the jugular vein and the femoral artery. Note their locations in Figures 6–6 and 6–7, respectively.

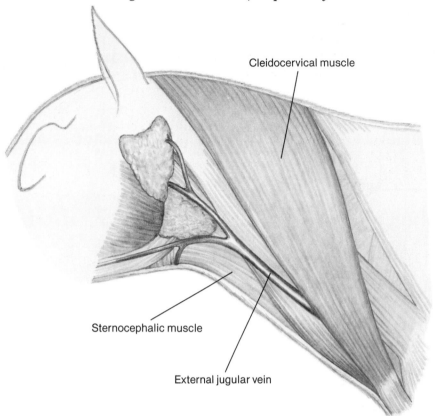

Cleidocervical muscle

Sternocephalic muscle

External jugular vein

Figure 6–6. Location of the external jugular vein within the neck (left view, after removal of the cutaneous muscles).

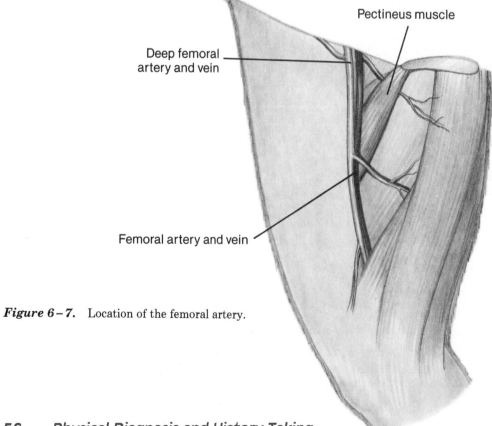

Pectineus muscle

Deep femoral artery and vein

Femoral artery and vein

Figure 6–7. Location of the femoral artery.

Observation

The pattern of respirations should be observed. Are there positional changes in the respiratory pattern? Is the animal coughing during the examination? Examine the area of the jugular groove. This is not always possible in long-haired pets, but if the animal is calm, a jugular pulse may be visible even under long hair. Note the extent of the jugular pulsations with the animal in various positions. Observe the shape of the chest and its symmetry. Note the position of the apex beat if visible. Note the color of the mucous membranes and the capillary refill time, assessment of which is made by using a fingertip to blanch an area of buccal mucosa and then measuring the time until the normal color returns.

Dyspnea often occurs when an animal that has pulmonary edema or pleural effusion secondary to heart disease lies in lateral recumbency.

A jugular pulse when the animal is in an upright position is suggestive of right heart failure.

Cardiomegaly results in a displacement of the apex beat.

A capillary refill time greater than 2.0 seconds suggests cardiovascular compromise.

Palpation

Palpate the chest wall and locate the apex beat (see Fig. 6–5). In addition, note any abnormal vibrations transmitted through the thoracic wall. Palpate the femoral pulse, noting its intensity, rhythm, and rate (Fig. 6–8). Pulse pressures are depicted in Figure 6–9. Palpate the limbs and the abdomen, noting any edema or ascites, respectively. Palpate over the area of the carotid artery and note any vibrations.

Palpable thrills, or vibrations, are felt with cardiac murmurs of grade 5 or higher.

Figure 6–9 illustrates characteristic pulse pressure types and their associated conditions.

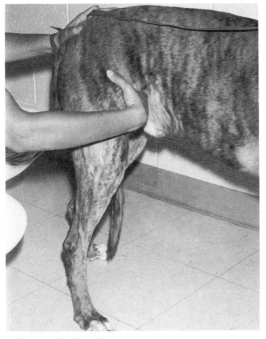

Figure 6–8. Palpation of the femoral pulse.

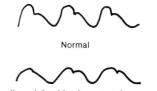

Normal

Small, weak (low blood pressure, low stroke volume, aortic stenosis, increased peripheral resistance)

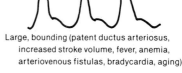

Large, bounding (patent ductus arteriosus, increased stroke volume, fever, anemia, arteriovenous fistulas, bradycardia, aging)

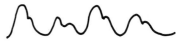

Bigeminal pulses (premature ventricular contractions)

Figure 6–9. Depiction of pulse pressures and the abnormalities associated with them.

Edema of the extremities or ventrum is indicative of poor peripheral circulation. Ascites is secondary to hepatic congestion associated with right heart failure.

Palpable thrills over the carotid arteries are associated with aortic stenosis.

Auscultation

With the bell portion of the stethoscope, listen to the various valve areas. What sounds should be heard?

1. Listen to the first heart sound (S1), attempting to block out the other heart sounds. Note the intensity and any splitting of the first sound. The first heart sound is usually longer and louder than the second heart sound (S2). It is heard best over the left apex area (fourth to sixth intercostal space to the left of the sternum). Increased intensity of S1 is normal during periods of increased sympathetic tone (exercise, excitement).

2. Listen to S2, attempting to disregard the other heart sounds. Note the intensity and any splitting. S2 is usually shorter, sharper, and higher pitched than S1. Normally, S2 is loudest over the left base (third to fourth intercostal space at the costochondral junction).

3. Listen for extra sounds during systole; then listen during diastole. Characterize the sounds.

Heart sounds may be difficult to hear in an animal with heavy muscling, excessive subcutaneous fat, long-hair coat, and fluid in the chest.

S2 may be accentuated by pulmonary hypertension, as in heartworm disease.

Adventitious cardiac sounds include murmurs, extra sounds, and splitting of sounds. A *murmur* is a prolonged series of audible vibrations that occurs during a normally silent part of the cardiac cycle. Murmurs should be characterized by their location, intensity (grade), timing within the cardiac cycle, duration, shape, and quality. The grading of cardiac murmurs follows:

GRADE 1   Heard after intent listening in a quiet room

GRADE 2   Quiet but readily heard when the stethoscope is placed on the chest

GRADE 3   A low to moderate intensity murmur

GRADE 4   A moderate intensity murmur heard on both sides of the chest

GRADE 5   A loud murmur with a palpable thrill

GRADE 6   A loud murmur with a palpable thrill that can be heard with the bell of the stethoscope removed from the chest wall

The timing of the murmur is helpful in localizing the source and nature of the problem. Figure 6–10 describes the various cardiac

The murmurs of mitral insufficiency and ventricular septal defects are holosystolic, whereas the murmurs of aortic and pulmonic stenosis are midsystolic and crescendo-decrescendo in configuration. Anemic and physiologic murmurs are usually early systolic. The murmur of a patent ductus arteriosus is holosystolic and holodiastolic.

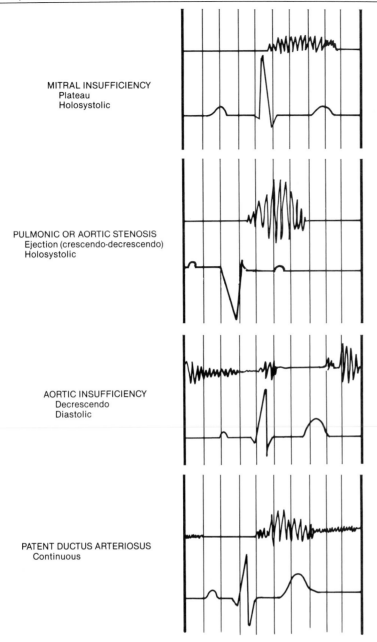

MITRAL INSUFFICIENCY
Plateau
Holosystolic

PULMONIC OR AORTIC STENOSIS
Ejection (crescendo-decrescendo)
Holosystolic

AORTIC INSUFFICIENCY
Decrescendo
Diastolic

PATENT DUCTUS ARTERIOSUS
Continuous

Figure 6-10. Shape and timing of selected cardiac murmurs.

murmurs and their timing within the cardiac cycle. Murmurs can be heard throughout systole (holosystolic) or may occur during only part of systole (midsystolic or late systolic). The same terminology can be used to describe diastolic murmurs.

The shape and quality of the murmur vary with the type of valvular abnormality. Ejection murmurs begin softly, increase in intensity to a peak, and then decrease in intensity again before ending. Regurgitant murmurs have a uniform intensity throughout and are termed plateau murmurs. Murmurs due to stenosis are characteristically harsh, whereas murmurs of insufficiency are usually high-pitched and blowing.

Other adventitious sounds include *gallop rhythms* and *splitting of heart sounds*. These sounds are of short duration. The third heart sound (S3) is not normally heard in dogs but can be heard if there is congestive heart failure or significant ventricular hypertrophy. It immediately follows S2 and is associated with rapid ventricular filling (Fig. 6–11). The fourth heart sound (S4), or the atrial sound, immediately precedes S1 (Fig. 6–11). It can be heard in dogs if atrioventricular heart block exists. Gallop rhythms are caused by the existence of the third or fourth heart sound. The three beats together, S1, S2, and S3 or S4, sound like the three-beat gait of a galloping horse. The presence of S3 is called a protodiastolic gallop rhythm. A presystolic gallop is caused by the presence of S4. The presence of both S3 and S4 heart sounds is designated a summation gallop.

The splitting of S1 can be caused by bundle branch blocks, especially of the right side, and ventricular extrasystoles. Splitting of S2 can occur with atrial septal defects, pulmonary hypertension, right to left shunting anomalies, right bundle branch block, and ventricular extrasystoles. Paradoxic splitting of S2 occurs with left bundle branch block and aortic stenosis. This splitting occurs on expiration rather than inspiration.

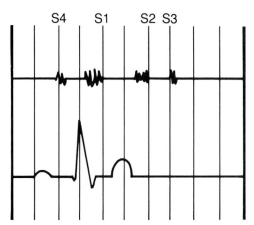

Figure 6–11.   Location of the third and fourth heart sounds within the cardiac cycle is illustrated.

Splitting of the heart sounds is a result of asynchronous closing of the valves. Splitting of S1 is a result of asynchronous closing of the atrioventricular valves. It can be normal in large and giant breed dogs.

"Clicks" are extra sounds that may be heard during auscultation of the heart. Ejection "clicks" are characterized by the accentuation of the terminal portion of S1. Systolic "clicks" occur during midsystole, are high-pitched, and may vary in intensity from beat to beat.

Pulmonic stenosis, aortic stenosis, atrial septal defects, and pulmonary hypertension are associated with ejection clicks. Systolic clicks can be heard with mitral insufficiency.

Consider the rate and rhythm of the heart. As you listen with your stethoscope, palpate the femoral artery. Do the pulses coincide with the heart sounds heard? Are pulses consistent in intensity?

Arrhythmias produce characteristic alterations in the heart sounds. Some have been mentioned above, but the most evident change is the variation in timing between the groups of heart sounds associated with each beat. When auscultating an arrhythmia, it is important to note the following:

1. The ventricular rate (bradycardia, normal, tachycardia)
2. The basic rhythm (if irregular, does it coincide with respiration?)
3. The intensity of the heart sounds
4. Splitting of the heart sounds
5. Absence of beats where they should occur
6. Extra sounds or premature beats

Heart sounds without a corresponding pulse are caused by premature contractions, especially ventricular in origin. Pulses of variable intensity are associated with changes in cardiac output, as seen with atrial fibrillation or ventricular tachycardia.

Figure 6–12 and Tables 6–1 and 6–2 illustrate the approach to the diagnosis of arrhythmias. Tachyarrhythmias are caused by atrial fibrillation, ventricular tachycardia, and sinus tachycardia. Bradyarrhythmias are caused by sinus bradycardia, sinus block, and second- and third-degree heart block. Unexpected pauses are caused by dropped beats, as in sinus block and atrioventricular block. Pronounced sinus arrhythmia may cause distinct pauses. In addition, compensatory pauses are common after premature contractions. Extra beats that seem to come early are a result of premature atrial, junctional, or ventricular contractions.

Sinus arrhythmia is a common, normal arrhythmia in dogs. It is characterized by an increased heart rate on inspiration and slowing of the heart rate during expiration.

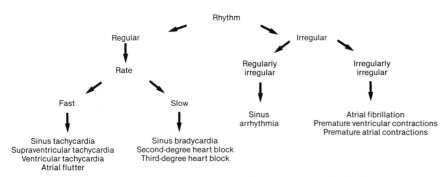

Figure 6–12. Algorithm for the diagnosis of arrhythmias.

Table 6-1
REGULAR ARRHYTHMIAS

Description	Usual Rate	Clinical Manifestations
Fast		
Sinus tachycardia	160-200 >220 (puppies) >240 (cats)	Normal heart sounds
Supraventricular tachycardia	>160 (medium-large breed dogs) >180 (toy breed dogs) >240 (cats)	Normal heart sounds
Atrial flutter with regular ventricular beats	>300 (dogs) >350 (cats)	Normal heart sounds
Ventricular tachycardia	>100 (dogs) >150 (cats)	Split S1, S2; S1 varies in intensity
Slow		
Sinus bradycardia	<70 (dogs) <160 (cats)	Normal heart sounds
Second-degree heart block	<70 (dogs) <160 (cats)	Atrial sound (S4) may be heard
Third-degree heart block	<40 (dogs) <60 (cats)	Variable intensity of heart sounds

Table 6-2
IRREGULAR ARRHYTHMIAS

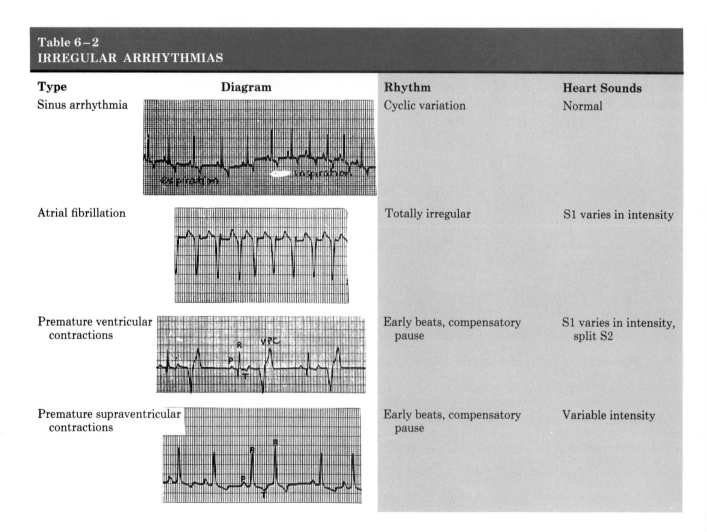

Type	Diagram	Rhythm	Heart Sounds
Sinus arrhythmia		Cyclic variation	Normal
Atrial fibrillation		Totally irregular	S1 varies in intensity
Premature ventricular contractions		Early beats, compensatory pause	S1 varies in intensity, split S2
Premature supraventricular contractions		Early beats, compensatory pause	Variable intensity

Percussion

Percussion of the heart involves two zones. These are (1) the area of absolute cardiac dullness that corresponds to the area of contact of the pericardium with the thoracic wall, and (2) the area of relative cardiac dullness. The area of absolute dullness is used to assess the heart for hypertrophy, displacement, or pericardial effusion. It is located on the left side from the sternum to the costochondral junctions of the fourth and fifth spaces and on the right side 1 to 2 cm from the sternum in the fourth and fifth spaces (Fig. 6–13). The area of relative dullness corresponds to the area of the heart underlying the lungs and is elicited by stronger percussion. It is difficult to hear in animals.

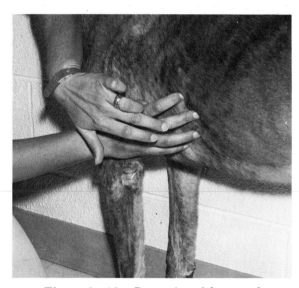

Figure 6–13. Percussion of the area of absolute cardiac dullness.

DIFFERENCES IN THE CAT

The heart is located between the fourth interspace and seventh rib in the cat. Owing to the small body size of cats, the valve areas are difficult to auscultate separately because the bell of the stethoscope lies over all three areas at once. The heart rate of the cat is rapid, and it is more difficult to detect adventitious sounds than in the dog.

Cats with hypertrophic cardiomyopathy often have protodiastolic gallops, whereas cats with dilatative cardiomyopathy often have presystolic gallops. Palpation of the femoral pulses in cats with cardiomyopathy may reveal decreased or absent pulses. This is associated with aortic thromboembolism and is characterized by cool limbs and cyanotic toenails. The skin over the legs is described as cardboard-like, and the cats have varying degrees of decreased motor function as well.

RECOMMENDED READING

1. Hahn AH: Examination of the cardiovascular system. Vet Clin North Am 11(3):481, 1981.
2. Evans HB, Christensen GC: Miller's Anatomy of the Dog, 2nd ed. Philadelphia, WB Saunders, 1979.
3. Kirk RW, Bistner SI: Handbook of Veterinary Procedures and Emergency Treatment, 3rd ed. Philadelphia, WB Saunders, 1981.
4. Smetzer DL: Auscultation of the heart. Class notes, University of Illinois, Urbana, IL, 1972.
5. Tilkian AG, Conover MB: Understanding Heart Sounds and Murmurs, 2nd ed. Philadelphia, WB Saunders, 1984.

Gastrointestinal System

APPLIED ANATOMY

The structures of the mouth and oral cavity have already been covered in Chapter 4. The esophagus travels down the neck and enters the thoracic cavity to the left of the trachea. It then courses through the thorax to the hiatus of the diaphragm.

The abdominal body wall consists of the skin, several layers of fascia and muscle, and the peritoneum (Fig. 7–1). From external to internal are the external abdominal oblique (fibers run caudoventrally), internal abdominal oblique (fibers run cranioventrally), rectus abdominis (along the ventral midline), and transversus abdominis muscles. The inguinal canal is an opening through the abdominal muscles. Its entrance is the superficial inguinal ring, which is a slit in the aponeurosis of the external abdominal oblique. The superficial inguinal lymph nodes lie over the origin of the pectineus muscle and drain the area of the mammae, scrotum, and ventral abdominal wall to the level of the umbilicus. The vasculature in this area includes the cranial and caudal superficial epigastric arteries and veins, which run parallel to each other on either side of the midline in the subcutaneous tissues. The costal arch marks the caudal extent of the bony thorax. Its rigidness prohibits palpation of the cranial abdominal viscera in most animals.

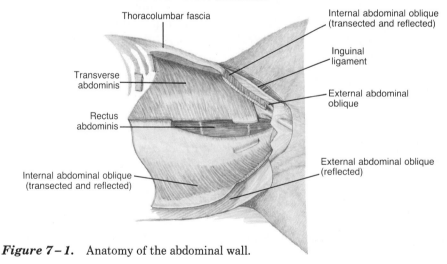

Figure 7–1. Anatomy of the abdominal wall.

The peritoneal cavity contains the organs of the digestive tract caudal to the eosphagus. It can be divided into quadrants for ease of structure localization. There are many ways to do this but perhaps the easiest is to designate cranial, middle, and caudal quadrants, which, when used to describe a structure, can be further subdivided into dorsal and ventral and/or left and right sections (Fig. 7–2). In the **cranial quadrant** lie the liver, stomach, the cranial duodenal

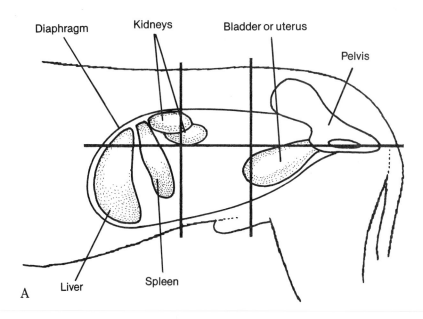

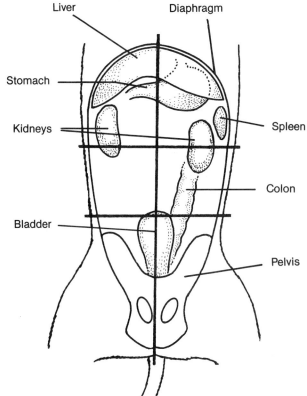

Figure 7–2. The abdomen can be divided into quadrants for ease of identifying abdominal organs or masses by palpation. *A,* lateral projection; *B,* ventrodorsal projection.

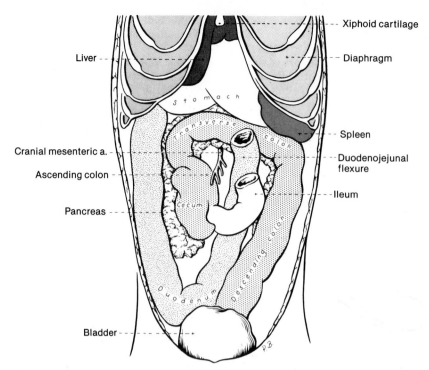

Xiphoid cartilage

Liver

Diaphragm

Spleen

Cranial mesenteric a.

Duodenojejunal
flexure

Ascending colon

Ileum

Pancreas

Bladder

Figure 7–3. The gastrointestinal organs present in the cranial abdominal quadrant include the stomach, liver, transverse colon, proximal duodenum, and pancreas. (Used by permission. From Evans HB, deLahunta A: Miller's Guide to the Dissection of the Dog. Philadelphia, WB Saunders, 1971.)

flexure and the initial third of the descending duodenum, the transverse colon, and the pancreas (Figs. 7–2 and 7–3). The liver rarely extends caudal to the costal arch in normal dogs. The stomach contacts the visceral surface of the liver. The location of the stomach is variable depending on the degree of distention (Figs. 7–2 to 7–4). The empty stomach lies within the costal arch caudal to the liver, between the planes of the ninth thoracic and first lumbar vertebrae. It lies parallel to the tenth intercostal space. The fundus of the stomach is to the left of the midline, the body of the stomach lies on the midline, and the pyloric part of the stomach extends to the right of the midline. When moderately full, the stomach expands to the left, touching the diaphragm caudal to the liver but not reaching the ventral abdominal wall. The greater curvature of the full stomach may lie transversely on the ventral abdominal wall halfway between the xiphoid process and the pubis (Fig. 7–4).

The duodenum is the most fixed part of the small intestine. It begins on the right side of the abdomen, where it receives food from the pyloric part of the stomach. After a short dorsocranial course, it becomes the descending duodenum, which courses down the right abdominal wall. The pancreas is composed of a body and right and left lobes. The body is located at the pyloroduodenal junction. The left lobe extends along the greater curvature of the stomach in the peritoneal layers that form the dorsal part of the omental bursa. The right lobe lies next to the descending duodenum within the meso-

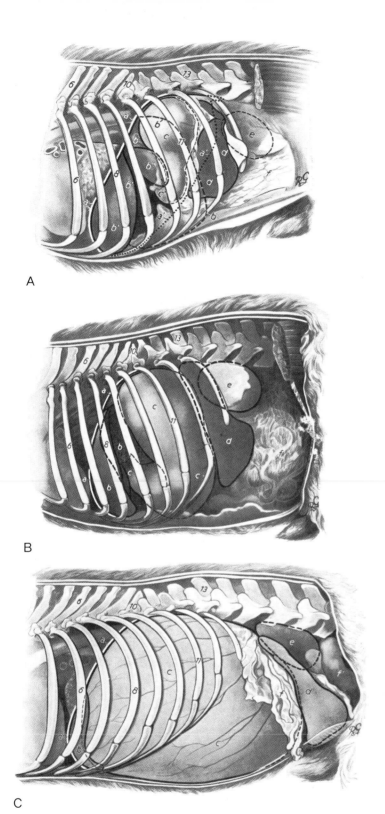

A

B

C

Figure 7–4. The variation in the caudal extent of the stomach depending on the degree of distention is shown. *A*, Stomach almost full. *B*, Stomach moderately full. *C*, Stomach greatly distended. *a* Diaphragm; *a'* Line of diaphragmatic attachment *(A)*; *b—b″* Liver, some of its outlines in heavy broken lines: *b* left lateral lobe (removed in *A* and *B*), *b'* left medial lobe (not visible in *C*), *b″* papillary process (visible only in *A*), *c* Stomach, some of its outlines in thin broken lines; *c'* Pylorus (not visible in *C*); *d* Spleen, some of its outlines in broken lines; *e* Left kidney, some of its outlines in broken lines; *f* Greater omentum; *f'* Jejunum *(C)*. *6, 10, 13* Thoracic vertebrae of like number; *6, 8, 11* Left ribs of like number. (Used by permission. From Nickel R, Schummer A, Sack WO: The Viscera of Domestic Mammals, 2nd ed, p 124. New York, Springer-Verlag, 1979.)

duodenum. The transverse colon lies in contact with the greater curvature of the stomach and travels across the midline from right to left.

The **middle quadrant** of the abdomen comprises the area between the planes of the second and fifth lumbar vertebrae. The greater curvature of the stomach, when full, may extend into this quadrant. Approximately the middle third of the descending duodenum with the associated portion of pancreas lies on the right side of the middle quadrant. The majority of the freely movable jejunum and ileum lie within this quadrant as well. On the right side, the ileum joins the colon at the ileocecocolic junction within the middle quadrant. The ascending colon and the proximal part of the descending colon also occupy a portion of this quadrant. The mesenteric lymph nodes lie within the mesentery along the vessels. Most of the mesenteric lymph nodes are contained within the middle quadrant.

The distal descending colon, rectum, and parts of the small intestine are present in the **caudal quadrant.** Lymph nodes of importance in this area are the external iliac lymph nodes, which lie under the fifth and sixth lumbar vertebrae. These may be palpable per rectum only if enlarged. The rectum is the terminal portion of the descending colon that lies within the pelvic canal. The rectum ends at the anus, which is the mucocutaneous junction surrounded by the internal and external anal sphincters. On either side of the anus are the anal sacs and their openings. These are covered in Chapter 10.

Observation

Examine the animal's face around the mouth as well as the oral cavity. Note any wetness, discoloration, or stickiness to the hair. Examine the neck near the thoracic inlet for distention of the esophagus (Fig. 7–5). Observe the animal's abdomen from a distance. What is the animal's general body condition? Is the abdomen distended? Is the abdomen symmetric? What is the animal's posture like? Examine the anal area, noting any redness, swelling, discharge, or diarrheic feces on the hair.

The hair around the mouth of a nauseous animal may be matted with vomitus or wet with saliva.

Esophageal dilatation can result in visible distention of the esophagus at the thoracic inlet, especially evident on expiration.

Chronic gastrointestinal diseases can lead to significant weight loss or emaciation.

Gastric dilatation results in cranial abdominal distention; ascites associated with protein-losing enteropathies results in general abdominal enlargement.

The posture depicted in Figure 7–6 can be seen in dogs with chronic gastrointestinal foreign bodies.

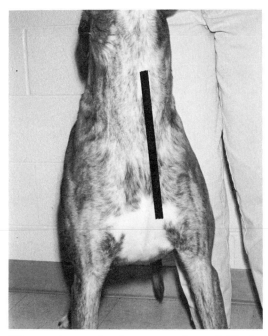

Figure 7–5. The area to examine for megaesophagus is illustrated by the black line.

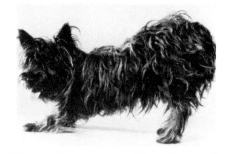

Figure 7–6. A dog with gastrointestinal pain may stand in the posture illustrated above. (Used by permission. From Sherding RG: Diseases of the small bowel. In Ettinger SJ: Textbook of Veterinary Internal Medicine, 2nd ed, p 1336. Philadelphia, WB Saunders, 1983.)

Palpation

Palpate the neck, feeling for distention of the esophagus at the thoracic inlet. Note any fluctuant swelling or crepitus.

Palpation of the abdomen is a skill that can be developed with patience and practice. Initially, palpate the animal in a standing position (Fig. 7–7). Later, it may be worthwhile to place the animal in other positions to clarify the presence or location of an abnormality. Begin with the dorsal cranial quadrant. Stand to one side of the animal. It is often easier to palpate the cranial portion of the abdomen with the animal facing away from you. With flat hands, use the fingers of each hand on opposite sides of the body to apply gentle

Raising the animal's chest above the level of the abdomen may allow palpation of cranial abdominal masses (Fig. 7–8).

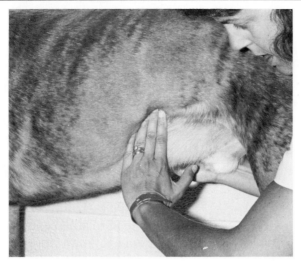

Figure 7–7. Two-handed technique of abdominal palpation.

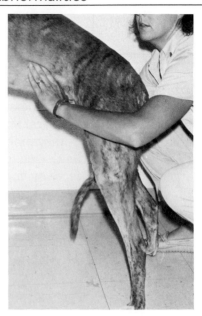

Figure 7–8. Palpation of a dog's abdomen with the chest elevated.

pressure medially until the two hands almost touch each other. This may be possible only in the relaxed pet that is not obese. As the fingers meet, move the hands ventrally, feeling the various internal structures slipping between your fingertips. This is referred to as a two-handed palpation technique and works well for most dogs. For small dogs, it is easier to use the one-handed technique. With the thumb on one side of the body and the four fingers on the other, gently apply pressure medially on the abdomen until the fingers meet the thumb. Again move the hand ventrally, feeling the internal structures slipping between the thumb and fingers. Repeat the same procedures for the middle and caudal quadrants.

Table 7–1 lists disorders of the gastrointestinal tract detectable by palpation and their associated conditions.

An enlarged liver may be palpated in the cranial abdominal quadrant just caudal to the costal arch. Generalized enlargement can be palpated on both sides ventrally. The edges feel rounded. Variable-sized nodules can be palpated on an asymmetrically enlarged liver. The unaffected edges of the liver may still be sharp.

An intussusception can be felt as a tubular structure with a firm consistency in the middle abdominal quadrant. Continuation of the intestines can be palpated at each end of the intussusception. Infiltrative or inflammatory bowel disease causes the intestines to feel thickened or more prominent as they slip through one's fingers.

Table 7-1
DISORDERS OF THE GASTROINTESTINAL TRACT AND ASSOCIATED FINDINGS

Disease	Abdominal Fluid	Pain	Palpation Findings
Gastric dilatation/volvulus	−	+ Generalized	Distention of cranial quadrant, tympanitic, enlarged spleen
Gastric neoplasia	±	−	± mass
Gastric foreign body	−	+	± mass
Gastroenteritis	−	±	Fluid ± gas-filled intestines
Infiltrative bowel disease	+ if low albumin	−	Thickened intestines, ascites, emaciation
Intestinal foreign body	+ if perforated	+	± mass, fluid
Intestinal neoplasia	±	+	± mass
Intussusception	±	+	± tubular mass, fluid
Megacolon	−	−	Tubular, doughy mass
Pancreatitis	±	+	Cranial abdominal pain
Pancreatic neoplasia	±	+	± mass
Hepatitis			
Acute	±	±	Enlarged liver, rounded edges
Chronic	+	−	Liver not palpable
Hepatic lipidosis	−	−	Enlarged liver, rounded edges
Hepatic neoplasia	±	±	Diffuse or nodular liver enlargement

If any abnormal structures are noted, describe them as to location, mobility, associated structures, consistency, size, shape, and presence or absence of pain. Note the presence of pain upon abdominal palpation and localize it if possible.

Palpate the inguinal lymph node, noting its size, shape, and consistency.

A digital rectal examination should be done to complete the examination of the gastrointestinal tract. Use an examination glove and lubricate one finger. Gently enter the rectum, noting the strength of the anal sphincter. As you advance your finger cranially, note any resistance or excessive pain. When you have advanced your finger as far as it will go, palpate 360 degrees around the rectum as you move your finger caudally. Note any enlargement of the external iliac lymph nodes dorsally. Are there any masses, ulceration, or diverticula? Does the rectum deviate to one side or the other? What is the consistency of the feces in the colon?

Pain can be associated with peritonitis, pancreatitis, intussusception, abscesses, or trauma.

Most dogs resent rectal palpation and anal tone should be high. Polyps are pedunculated masses of variable size that are attached to the colonic or rectal mucosa. Broad-based attachment of a mass suggests a more aggressive disease.

Perineal hernias cause a sac-like outpouching of the rectum to one or both sides of the anus. Often all that separates your finger from the outside is the skin and rectal mucosa (Fig. 7–9). Perianal fistulas appear as linear or circular ulcerated areas radiating around the anus.

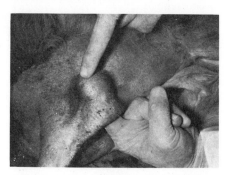

Figure 7–9. A perineal hernia is an outpouching of the rectum laterally through the weakened muscles of the pelvic diaphragm. The index finger of the left hand is inside the rectum pushing through the perineal hernia. (Courtesy of Dr. Howard Seim, Colorado State University.)

Auscultation

Although not used often in small animals, auscultation of the abdomen can be used to assess bowel motility. Most bowel sounds originate from the stomach, because the small and large intestinal sounds are brief. Bowel sounds are created by the movement of fluid and air. The presence of air increases the amplitude of the sounds in the stomach, whereas fluids increase the amplitude of the sounds in the small intestine. The rate of sound production varies in the normal animal depending on the phase of the digestive cycle occurring at that time; therefore, there is no specific number of sounds per minute that is considered normal. What may be important, however, is hearing no sound at all. This suggests ileus or total lack of motility. Continual gut sounds may be noted in some cases of hypermotility as well. Auscultation of a murmur within the abdomen may be indicative of an intra-abdominal arteriovenous shunt.

Percussion

The technique of percussion has been described (Chapter 5). The normal area of percussion of the liver is primarily on the right side along the entire basal border of the right lung to the costal arch (Fig. 7–10). On the left side, there is a small area of dullness in the seventh to ninth intercostal space. Percussion of a distended abdomen can help differentiate the presence of gas in the gastrointestinal tract or fluid in the peritoneal cavity.

Gastric dilatation causes a characteristic high-pitched tympanic sound on percussion. Ascites does not percuss well, but ballotement results in the visualization of a fluid wave.

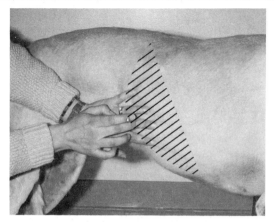

Figure 7–10. Normal area of hepatic percussion.

DIFFERENCES IN THE CAT

Always remember to examine under the tongue for a string foreign body. The technique is described in Chapter 4. Palpation of the abdomen in the cat is much easier than in the dog because the body wall is relaxed and internal organs are readily felt, especially the kidneys and urinary bladder. One-handed palpation is usually the preferable technique (Fig. 7–11). Anatomically, the cat's entire stomach is to the left of the midline, although this changes somewhat with the degree of distention. Rectal palpation is not routinely done in the cat owing to the small size of the rectum.

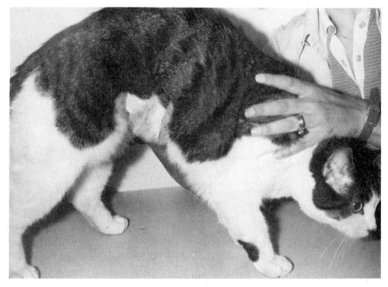

Figure 7–11. One-handed abdominal palpation technique being utilized in a cat.

RECOMMENDED READINGS

1. Evans HB, Christensen GC: Miller's Anatomy of the Dog, 2nd ed. Philadelphia, WB Saunders, 1979.
2. Strombeck DR: Small Animal Gastroenterology. Davis, CA, Stonegate Publishing, 1979.
3. Zimmer JF: Examination of the gastrointestinal system. Vet Clin North Am 11(3):561, 1981.

Genitourinary Tract

ELLEN M. POFFENBARGER

APPLIED ANATOMY

Female Dog

The vulva is formed by the two labia that surround the external urogenital orifice. Within the vulva is the vestibule. On the ventral floor of the vestibule is the clitoral fossa, which contains the clitoris. The urethral papilla lies on the floor at the junction of the vestibule and vagina. The urethra opens on this papilla at the level of the ischial arch (Fig. 8–1). The vagina is anterior to the vestibule and dorsal to the urethra. It is characterized by its longitudinal mucosal folds. The cervix marks the cranial extent of the vagina and the opening into the bicornuate uterus. The uterine horns travel cranially from the body of the uterus in the pelvic canal to the caudal poles of their respective kidneys. The urethra passes through the pelvic canal from its external orifice on the urethral papilla to the bladder. Within the caudal abdomen, from dorsal to ventral, lie the descending colon, uterus, and urinary bladder. With distention, the uterine horns may lie below the bladder on the floor of the abdomen.

Male Dog

The scrotum is divided into two cavities by a median septum. Each cavity contains a testis, an epididymis, and the distal portion of the spermatic cord. The head of the epididymis is located on the craniolateral aspect of each testicle. This structure is continued as the body of the epididymis along the dorsolateral aspect of the testicle and ends as the tail of the epididymis, which courses medially to become the ductus deferens within the spermatic cord (Fig. 8–2). Beginning distally, within the prepuce, is the glans penis. The distal part is referred to as the pars longa glandis; the proximal part is called the bulbus glandis. The bulbus glandis is composed of highly vascular tissue that expands upon erection to anchor the penis within the vagina during copulation. The os penis is a long bone that lies within the glans penis. It is grooved ventrally to house the penile

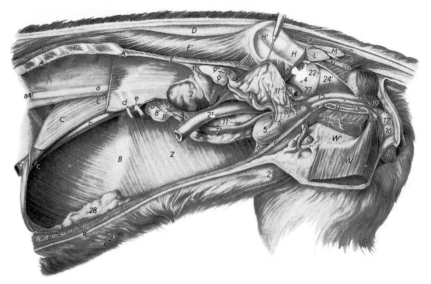

Figure 8–1. Female dog urogenital anatomy. *A*, Tenth rib. *A'*, Thirteenth rib. *B*, Right costal arch. *B'*, Left tenth costal cartilage. *C*, Left crus of diaphragm. *C'*, *C''*, Right crus of diaphragm. *C'''*, Costal part of diaphragm. *D*, Longissimus. *E*, *E'*, Iliocostalis. *F*, *F'*, Ext. intercostal muscles. *G*, Int. abdominal oblique. *H*, *H'*, Ilium. *J*, Caudal part of sartorius. *K*, Iliopsoas. *L*, Gluteus medius. *M*, Gluteus supf. *N*, Sacrotuberous ligament. *O*, Sacrocaudalis dorsalis lateralis. *P*, Intertransversarius dorsalis. *Q*, Sacrocaudalis ventralis lateralis. *R*, Coccygeus. *S*, Levator ani. *T*, Obturator int. *U*, Floor of pelvis. *V*, Adductor magnus et brevis. *W*, Gracilis. *W'*, Symphysial tendon. *X*, *Y*, Rectus abdominis. *Z*, Right transversus abdominis, covered with transverse fascia and peritoneum. *Z'*, Origin of left transversus abdominis.

a, Aorta. *b*, Caudal vena cava. *c*, Stump of hepatic veins as they enter the caudal vena cava. *d*, Celiac artery. *e*, Cranial mesenteric artery. *f*, Ischiatic nerve. *g*, Femoral artery and vein. *h*, Ext. pudendal vein. *i*, Supf. inguinal lymph nodes.

1, Right kidney. *2*, Left kidney. *2'*, Hilus of left kidney. *4*, Left ureter, visible through lateral lig. of bladder. *5*, Urinary bladder. *6*, Left lateral lig. of bladder. *6'*, Round lig. of bladder (degenerated umbilical artery). *6''*, Median lig. of bladder. *7*, Urethra. *7''*, Level of ext. urethral opening. *8*, Position of right ovary. *8'*, Fat-filled mesosalpinx. *8''*, Entrance to ovarian bursa. *9*, Position of left ovary. *9'*, Fat-filled mesosalpinx. *9''*, Fat-free area in mesosalpinx. *10*, Right uterine tube. *11*, Mesometrium. *11'*, Mesovarium. *11''*, Suspensory lig. of ovary. *11'''*, Round lig. of uterus. *11''''*, Vaginal ring. *12*, Right uterine horn. *13*, Left uterine horn. *14*, Body of uterus. *15*, Vagina. *16*, Vestibule. *17'*, Vestibular bulb. *18*, Vulva. *18'*, Body of clitoris. *18''*, Left crus clitoridis, transected. *19*, Constrictor vulvae. *20*, Mesocolon. *21*, Descending colon. *22*, Pelvic fascia and parietal peritoneum, fenestrated to expose rectum. *24*, Rectum, covered with peritoneum. *24'*, Retroperitoneal part of rectum. *26*, Ext. anal sphincter. *27*, Teat of mammary gland. *28*, Fat-filled part of falciform ligament. *29*, Falciform ligament. (Used by permission. From Nickel R, Schummer A, Sack WO: The Viscera of Domestic Mammals, 2nd ed, p 373. New York, Springer-Verlag, 1973.)

urethra. Proximal to the glans penis is the body of the penis, which lies deep to the scrotum. The penile urethra continues through this portion of the penis surrounded by corpora cavernosa and spongiosa. At the level of the ischial arch, the pelvic urethra begins. The urethra continues through the prostrate gland as the prostatic urethra and ends at the urinary bladder. The spermatic cord enters the abdominal cavity through the inguinal canal.

The kidneys of the dog are retroperitoneal on either side of the aorta and caudal vena cava. The right kidney lies opposite the first three lumbar vertebrae, whereas the left kidney is slightly more caudal opposite the second, third, and fourth lumbar vertebrae. The right kidney is situated almost entirely under the ribs. The ureters travel on either side of the midline dorsally from the renal penis to the dorsocaudal (trigone) area of the bladder.

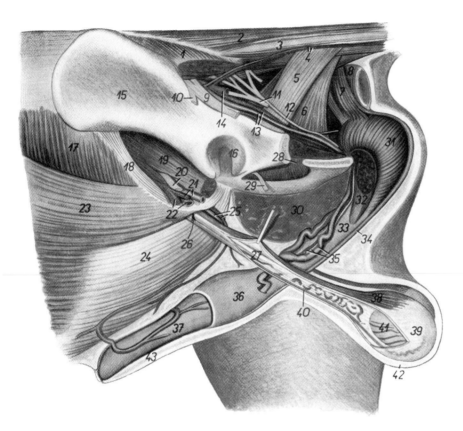

1. Superficial gluteal muscle
2. Lateral dorsal sacrococcygeal muscle
3. Intertransverse muscle of tail
4. Lateral artery and vein of tail
5. (Lateral) coccygeal muscle
6. Levator ani (medial coccygeal) muscle
7. External anal sphincter muscle (cranial portion)
8. External anal sphincter muscle (caudal portion)
9. Ischiadic nerve
10. Cranial gluteal nerve
11. Caudal cutaneous femoral nerve
12. Pudendal nerve
13. Internal pudendal artery and vein (visceral branch of internal iliac artery)
14. Internal iliac artery (parietal branch)
15. Wing of ilium
16. Acetabulum
17. Internal abdominal oblique muscle
18. Inguinal ligament
19. Iliopsoas muscle
20. Femoral nerve
21. Deep femoral artery and vein
22. Femoral artery and vein
23., 24. External abdominal oblique muscle
23. Lateral crus of external abdominal oblique muscle
24. Medial crus of external abdominal oblique muscle
25. External pudendal artery and vein
26. Inguinal canal
27. Spermatic cord
28. Internal obturator muscle
29. Obturator nerve
30. Adductor and gracilis muscles
31. Bulbospongiosus muscle
32. Ischiocavernous muscle
33. Body of penis
34. Retractor muscle of penis
35. Dorsal artery and vein of penis, dorsal nerve of penis
36. Bulbus glandis
37. Pars longa glandis
38. Cremaster muscle
39. Vaginal tunic and spermatic fascia
40. Ductus deferens
41. Testis
42. Scrotum
43. Preputium

Figure 8–2. Anatomy of the male dog's urogenital system. (Used by permission. From Popesko P: Atlas of Topographical Anatomy of the Domestic Animals, 2nd ed. Vol 3, p 186. Philadelphia, WB Saunders, 1977.)

Observation

Examine the vulvar area of the female dog and note any discharge, redness, swelling, or masses. What is the conformation of the vulva? Is the vulva covered by a dorsal fold of skin? Inspect the skin surrounding the vulva. In the male, inspect the prepuce for discharge, redness, swelling, or masses. Gently push the prepuce caudally and examine the penis for abnormalities. Note any dripping of urine from the vulva or penis. Does the animal make frequent attempts to urinate while in the examination room? Examine the scrotum for evidence of swelling, redness, or ulceration.

Estrus causes enlargement of the vulva and the presence of a vaginal discharge that may be sanguinous or mucoid depending on the phase of the cycle that is occurring. Pyometra or metritis is indicated by a purulent discharge from the vulva. Masses protruding from the vulva could include vaginal edema (Fig. 8–3), placenta or puppy, vaginal neoplasia, uterine prolapse, or clitoral hypertrophy (Fig. 8–4). Vulvar

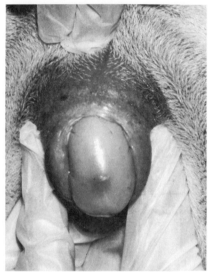

Figure 8–3. Mass protruding from this dog's vulva is characteristic of vaginal edema. (Courtesy of Dr. Patty Olson, Colorado State University.)

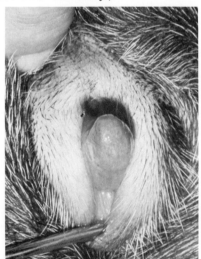

Figure 8–4. Enlarged clitoris can be seen emerging from this dog's vulva. (Courtesy of Dr. Patty Olson, Colorado State University.)

dermatitis is common in over-weight female dogs with proportionately small vulvas (Fig. 8–5).

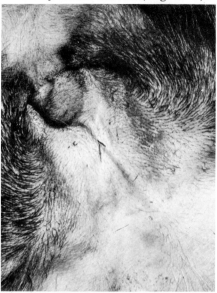

Figure 8–5. Vulvar dermatitis can be seen in the perivulvar skin of this dog. Note the "tucked up" appearance to the vulva. (Courtesy of Dr. Patty Olson, Colorado State University.)

Penile discharge can be indicative of prostatic disease; a bloody discharge from the prepuce can be observed with cystic hyperplasia of the prostate. Balanoposthitis may give rise to purulent preputial discharge. A persistent penile frenulum is a band of mucosa along the ventral surface of the penis that deviates the penis ventrally (Fig. 8–6). A roughened or nodular appearance of the penis suggests neoplasia.

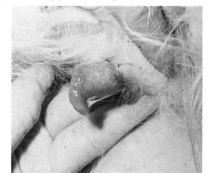

Figure 8–6. Abnormal band of tissue on the ventral aspect of the penis is termed a persistent penile frenulum. (Courtesy of Dr. Shirley Johnston, University of Minnesota.)

Dripping of urine from the vulva or penis is indicative of urinary incontinence. Pollakiuria (frequent attempts to urinate) is suggestive of lower urinary tract disease such as cystitis, urethritis, bladder stones, or bladder neoplasms.

Palpation

Palpate the abdomen in the dorsal portion of the cranial quadrant for the kidneys. The right kidney is usually not palpable in the dog; however, the left kidney, being more caudal and more freely movable, can be palpated in some dogs. Moving to the middle quadrant, the uterine horns may be palpated if enlarged due to pregnancy, infection, or fluid. In the caudal abdomen, the cervix and body of the uterus can be felt dorsal to the urinary bladder and ventral to the descending colon. In the male dog, palpate the caudal abdomen for the presence of the prostate gland. It can be located just caudal to the urinary bladder within the abdominal cavity if it is enlarged. The ease of urinary bladder palpation varies with its degree of distention. Very small and very large bladders are often difficult to feel. A moderately sized bladder is usually palpable in the caudal abdominal quadrant as a smooth pear-shaped structure that can vary from turgid to flaccid.

Enlargement of one or both kidneys may allow easy palpation of these structures. Kidneys can be larger than normal because of infectious, neoplastic, or anomalous conditions.

An enlarged uterus can be palpated as a doughy, tubular structure on the floor of the abdomen in the case of pyometra. Fetal vesicles or puppies may be palpated if the bitch is pregnant. Fetal vesicles feel like turgid, fluid-filled spheres. Fetuses are firmer and more irregular.

Pain on palpation of the caudal abdomen may be indicative of prostatitis, uterine stump granuloma, or bladder stones. Dogs with bladder calculi often have very small, firm bladders as a result of inflammation. The stones can sometimes be palpated in a relaxed animal.

Palpate the scrotum for the presence of two testicles of equal size and consistency. Note any pain, swelling, asymmetry, or change in consistency of the testes.

Testicular neoplasia is seen in older, intact male dogs and is detected by palpation of nodular mass(es) within the testicle. In certain breeds of dogs, cryptorchidism is common and results in the inability to palpate one or both testicles. Orchitis due to a variety of causes can lead to painful swelling of the testicles.

Rectal palpation should be completed on any male dog over 2 years of age or any dog exhibiting signs of lower urinary tract disease, especially if not neutered. On the floor of the pelvis, the tubular urethra can be identified. Within the pelvic canal, usually at the cranial aspect, the bilobed prostate gland can be felt. It is small in the neutered dog. Note any asymmetry, pain, masses, or firm areas. In some dogs, it is necessary to palpate the caudal abdomen with one hand while you palpate rectally with the other hand. With the hand palpating the abdomen, push the prostate gland dorsocaudally until it can be palpated with the finger of the other hand (Fig. 8–7).

The prostate is symmetrically enlarged and nonpainful in dogs with benign prostatic hypertrophy. Asymmetric enlargement of the prostate is consistent with neoplasia or prostatic cysts. Pain is usually associated with acute prostatitis.

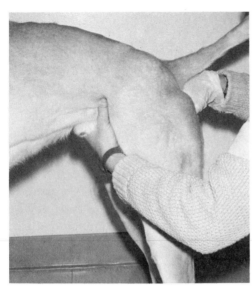

Figure 8–7.   Two-handed technique of prostate palpation allows palpation of some enlarged prostates that have migrated over the pelvic brim.

Vaginal strictures can be present at the vestibulovaginal or vestibulovulvar junction (Fig. 8–8). Vertical septa may also be palpated at the vestibulovaginal junction.

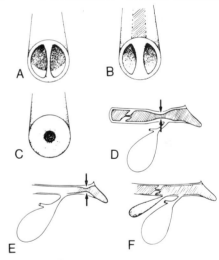

A rectal examination can be used to assess the intrapelvic portion of the urethra in females. The normal urethra is a tubular structure on the floor of the pelvis. A digital vaginal examination can be done to assess the vestibule, vagina, and urethral orifice. Gently advance a clean gloved and lubricated finger into the vestibule and over the ischial arch. The urethral papilla is a small protuberance on the ventral aspect at the vestibulovaginal junction. Note any asymmetry, pain, masses, or strictures. Does this area bleed easily?

Note: These examinations in the female are usually reserved for those animals that have historical abnormalities suggestive of lower urinary tract disease.

Figure 8–8.   Congenital anomalies of the vagina and vulva.
A, Vertical septum at the vestibulovaginal junction. *B,* Incomplete fusion of the müllerian ducts partitioning the vagina. *C,* Annular stricture at the vestibulovaginal junction. *D,* Hypoplasia of vestibulovaginal junction. *E,* Stenosis at vestibulovulvar junction. *F,* Secondary vaginal pouch (double vagina). (Used by permission. From Wykes PM, Soderberg SF: Congenital abnormalities of the canine vagina and vulva. J Am Anim Hosp Assoc 19:995, 1983.)

Auscultation and Percussion

Not readily applicable to this system.

DIFFERENCES IN THE CAT

The anatomic differences in the cat concern the location of the kidneys and the structure of the penis primarily. The kidneys are very freely movable in the cat and may be mistaken for abnormal masslike structures. The right kidney lies ventral to the first through the fourth lumbar vertebral transverse processes, and the left kidney lies ventral to the second through the fifth lumbar vertebral transverse processes. Both are readily palpable in all but the most obese cats. The size, location, consistency, and surface texture should be noted.

Renomegaly in cats is often the result of lymphosarcoma or polycystic renal disease. Small, irregular kidneys can be palpated in cats with chronic renal failure.

The penis of the male cat is structurally similar to the dog's; however, its orientation is unusual. The penis is directed caudoventrally and the urethral orifice opens caudodorsally (Fig. 8–9). It therefore does not make the arc as in the male dog. The cat's penis has spines at sexual maturity.

Urethral obstruction is common in male cats, and the "plugs" are often seen protruding from the urethral orifice (Fig. 8–10).

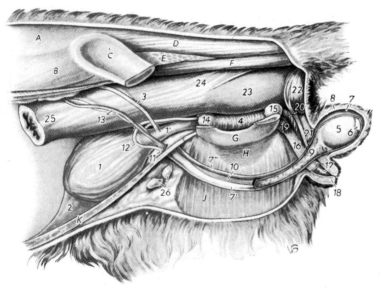

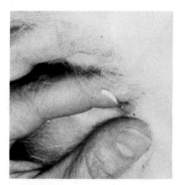

Figure 8–10. A urethral plug can be seen at the opening of the penile urethra.

Figure 8–9. Anatomy of the male cat's urogenital system. Left lateral aspect. *A*, Longissimus. *B*, Iliocostalis. *C*, Wing of ilium. *D*, Sacrocaudalis dorsalis lateralis. *E*, Gluteus supf. *F*, Sacrocaudalis ventralis lateralis. *G*, Floor of pelvis. *H*, Symphysial tendon, origin of adductor and gracilis muscles. *J*, Right gracilis. *K*, Ventral abdominal wall. *1*, Urinary bladder. *1'*, Neck of bladder. *2*, Median lig. of bladder. *3*, Left ureter. *4*, Pelvic part of urethra, surrounded by urethralis. *5*, Left testis. *6*, Tail of epididymis. *7,7'*, Left tunica vaginalis parietalis, its distal part fenestrated. *7"*, Proximal part of right tunica vaginalis parietalis. *8*, Scrotum. *9*, Spermatic cord. *10*, Cremaster. *11*, Vaginal ring. *12*, Left ductus deferens. *13*, Testicular artery and vein. *14*, Prostate gland. *15*, Bulbourethral gland. *16*, Penis. *17*, Free part of penis. *18*, Prepuce. *19*, Ischiocavernosus. *20*, Bulbospongiosus. *21*, Retractor penis. *22*, Ext. anal sphincter. *23*, Rectum. *24*, Rectococcygeus. *25*, Descending colon. *26*, Supf. inguinal lymph nodes. (Used by permission. From Nickel R, Schummer A, Sack WO: The Viscera of the Domestic Mammals, 2nd ed. New York, Springer-Verlag, 1973.)

A lack of penile spines in an intact male cat suggests the absence of hormonal influence. This may be a significant finding in the infertile male.

The urinary bladder of the cat is more spheric in shape than that of the dog and lies slightly more cranially within the abdomen. When palpating the cat's bladder, note particularly its size and consistency.

Rectal examinations are not usually performed in the cat.

Idiopathic feline lower urinary tract disease is a frequent reason that cats are presented for examination. Male cats with urethral obstruction have a very firm, distended bladder of variable size. Females and unobstructed males with lower urinary tract disease have small, painful bladders.

RECOMMENDED READINGS

1. Evans HB, Christensen GC: Miller's Anatomy of the Dog, 2nd ed. Philadelphia, WB Saunders, 1979.
2. Johnston SD: Examination of the genital system. Vet Clin North Am 11(3):543, 1981.
3. Popesko P: Atlas of Topographical Anatomy of Domestic Animals, 2nd ed. Philadelphia, WB Saunders, 1977.
4. Schummer A, Nickel R, Sack WO: The Viscera of Domestic Mammals. New York, Springer-Verlag, 1979.
5. Wykes PM, Soderberg SF: Congenital abnormalities of the canine vagina and vulva. J Am Anim Hosp Assoc 19:995, 1983.

Musculoskeletal System

APPLIED ANATOMY

This section reviews the structure and function of joints briefly and describes the landmarks of clinically important components of the musculoskeletal system.

Structure and Function of Joints

The most freely movable joints are the *synovial joints,* or diarthroses. All synovial joints are composed of a joint space, articular cartilage, joint fluid, and a joint capsule (Fig. 9–1). Depending on their function, some synovial joints have modifications such as menisci, fat pads, and intra-articular ligaments.

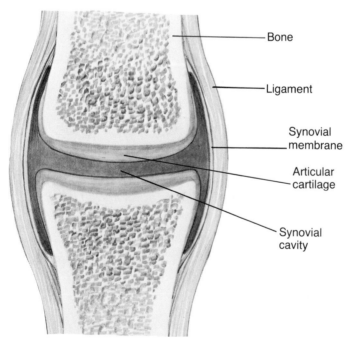

Figure 9–1. Basic structure of a synovial joint.

The *joint capsule* consists of a fibrous layer and a synovial membrane. The synovial membrane lines the joint space and covers the intra-articular ligaments, nerves, vessels, and muscles. It blends with the periosteum as it reflects onto the bone. The fibrous layer is thin and loose in the plane of joint motion but thickens to form collateral ligaments on the sides of the joint that move the least. The synovial membrane produces the synovial fluid, which lubricates the joint and nourishes the cartilage. It is a dialysate of plasma to which mucin has been added by the synovial cells. Hyaline cartilage covers the articular surfaces of the bones, providing a glasslike smoothness to the joint surface.

Menisci are fibrocartilaginous plates that absorb shock and distribute synovial fluid within the joint. They are present in the stifle and temporomandibular joints of dogs. *Ligaments,* or collagenous bands of tissue that attach bone to bone, maintain the structure and stability of most joints.

Fibrous joints and *cartilage joints* represent the two other types of articulations recognized in the dog and cat. These joints are relatively immobile. Fibrous joints are exemplified by the sutures of the cranium or the syndesmoses of the hyoid apparatus. Hyaline cartilage joints and fibrocartilaginous joints are the two types of cartilage joints, or synchondroses. In the growing animal, hyaline cartilage unites the epiphysis and diaphysis of long bones. As the bone matures, ossification occurs and growth stops. Fibrocartilaginous joints are illustrated by the pelvic and mandibular symphyses.

Synovial joints can be classified by the shape of the articular surface. The seven basic types are listed in Table 9–1.

Table 9–1
TYPES OF SYNOVIAL JOINTS

Type	Shape of Surface	Example
Plane	Flat	Costotransverse joint
Ball-and-socket	Convex, hemispheric head fitting into a concave structure	Hip, shoulder
Ellipsoidal	Convex elliptic surface fitting into concave elliptic surface	Radiocarpal
Hinge	Movable concave surface glides over a grooved convex surface	Humeroulnar
Condylar	Rounded prominences fit into reciprocal depressions	Stifle
Trochoid	Flat to slightly convex fitting into flat to slightly concave	Radioulnar
Saddle	Opposed surfaces, each of which is concave in one direction and convex in the other direction, usually at right angles	Interphalangeal

The movements of synovial joints are a result of the contraction of muscles that cross the joints (active movement) or the forces of gravity (passive movement). *Flexion* is the movement of two bones such that the angle between them becomes less than 180 degrees. Movement of two bones in relation to each other such that the angle approaches 180 degrees is referred to as *extension*. *Adduction* is the movement of a bone toward the median plane, whereas *abduction* is the opposite of this. When a limb follows the shape of a cone, the motion is referred to as *circumduction*. *Rotation* is the movement of a bone around its longitudinal axis.

Specific Joints

The temporomandibular joint is located just below the caudal aspect of the zygomatic arch (Fig. 9–2). The muscles of mastication are the temporalis muscles arising from the temporal fossae, the masseter muscles arising from the zygomatic arch, the pterygoid muscles arising from the pterygopalatine fossa, and the digastricus arising from the jugular process of the occipital bone.

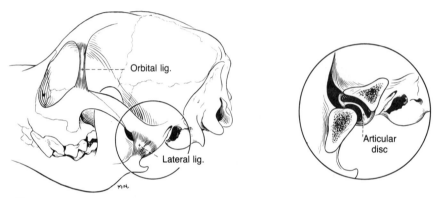

Figure 9–2. Temporomandibular joint of the dog is a synovial joint that has a meniscus. (Used by permission. From Evans HB, Christensen GC: Miller's Anatomy of the Dog, 2nd ed. Philadelphia, WB Saunders, 1979.)

The landmarks of the shoulder joint are the acromion of the scapula, which is on the lateral aspect of the proximal front leg at the level of the thoracic inlet, and the greater tubercle of the humerus, which is the most cranial bony prominence in the front limb (Fig. 9–3). The deltoideus muscle originates on the acromium, and the biceps brachii originates on the supraglenoid tubercle of the scapula. The tendon of the biceps travels medial to the greater tubercle of the humerus.

Medial to the shoulder joint lie the axillary artery and vein and the brachial plexus.

The elbow joint is a composite joint made up of the humeroulnar, humeroradial, and proximal radioulnar joints (Fig. 9–4). The joint space surrounds the humeral condyles in a crescent fashion. Flexion of the elbow joint opens the joint space caudally in the area of the olecranon fossa.

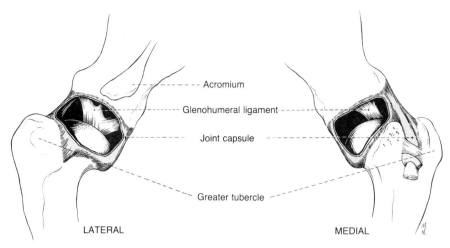

Figure 9-3. Shoulder joint of the dog. (Used by permission. From Evans HB, Christensen GC: Miller's Anatomy of the Dog, 2nd ed. Philadelphia, WB Saunders, 1979.)

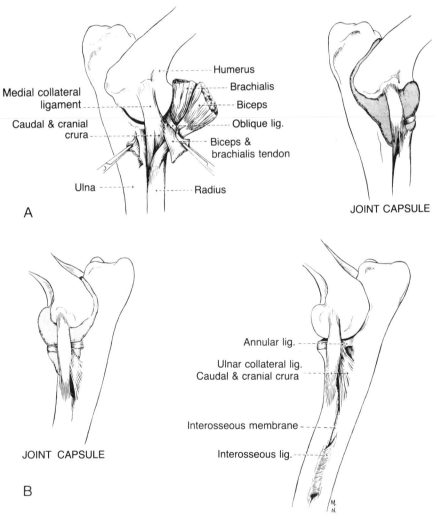

Figure 9-4. Elbow joint of the dog. *A*, Medial and *B*, lateral aspects. (Used by permission. From Evans HB, Christensen GC: Miller's Anatomy of the Dog, 2nd ed. Philadelphia, WB Saunders, 1979.)

The cephalic vein crosses the elbow joint superficially on its anterior surface.

The carpus is a combination of several articulations, including the antebrachiocarpal, the middle carpal, and the carpometacarpal joints (Fig. 9–5). Of the three carpal joints, the proximal antebrachiocarpal joint is capable of the most motion. It is a wedge-shaped joint when flexed. The sharp edge of the radius can be palpated on the dorsal aspect of the distal forearm. From medial to lateral, three tendons can be identified as they travel over the joint space: the extensor carpi radialis, the common digital extensor, and the lateral digital extensor. The accessory carpal bone is easily palpated on the caudolateral aspect of the carpus at the level of the antebrachiocarpal joint. The flexor carpi ulnaris inserts on the accessory carpal bone. The carpal canal runs medial to the accessory carpal bone on the caudal aspect of the carpus. Within the carpal canal are the tendons, nerves, arteries, and veins of the paw. The middle carpal joint is opened a small amount during flexion of the carpus; however, the carpometacarpal joint is relatively stationary.

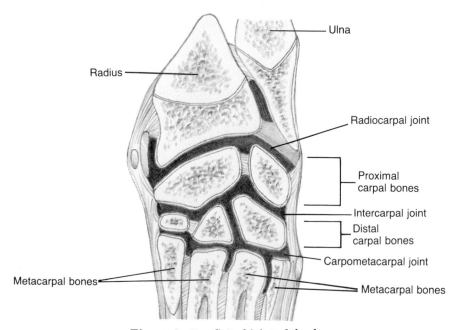

Figure 9–5. Carpal joint of the dog.

The accessory cephalic vein is visible as it crosses the central dorsal aspect of the carpal joint. The cephalic vein courses along the craniomedial surface of the joint.

The coxofemoral joint can be located by first finding the greater trochanter of the femur. The joint space is craniomedial to this prominence (Fig. 9–6). The caudal thigh muscles (biceps femoris, semitendinosus, and semimembranosus) originate on the ischiatic tuberosity and pass caudal to the greater trochanter. Of importance is the location of the sciatic nerve, which travels deep to the gluteal muscles proximal to the greater trochanter of the femur and then courses distally caudal to the greater trochanter between the biceps femoris and the semitendinosus muscles (Fig. 9–7).

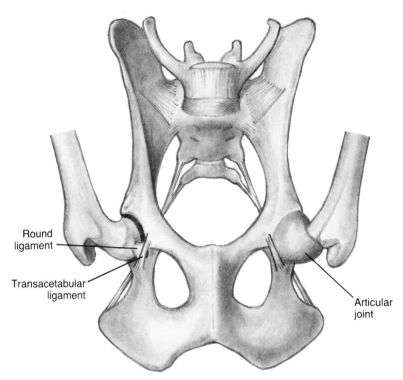

Figure 9 – 6. Coxofemoral joint of the dog.

Round ligament

Transacetabular ligament

Articular joint

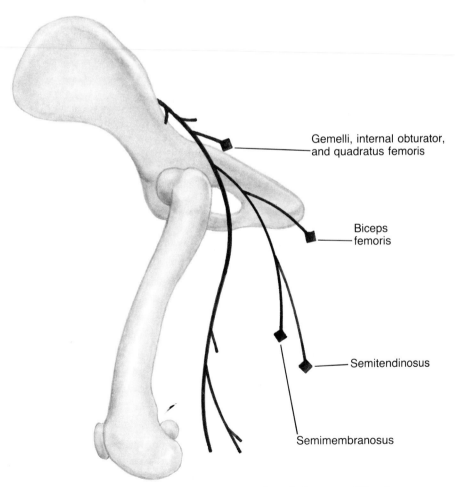

Figure 9 – 7. Anatomic location of the sciatic nerve of the dog.

Gemelli, internal obturator, and quadratus femoris

Biceps femoris

Semitendinosus

Semimembranosus

The landmarks of the stifle joint are the trochlear groove of the distal femur, tibial tuberosity, patellar tendon, and patella (Fig. 9–8). The patella should remain in the trochlear groove throughout the range of motion of the stifle joint. The joint capsule of the stifle is the largest in the body. It has three compartments, all of which freely communicate: the medial femorotibial, the lateral femorotibial, and the femoropatellar joints. There are medial and lateral menisci within the stifle joint.

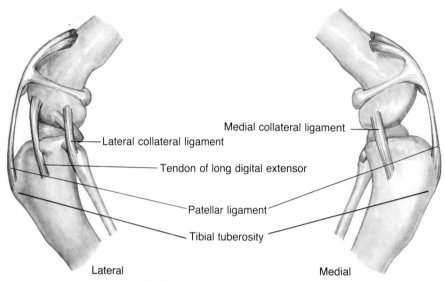

Medial collateral ligament

Lateral collateral ligament

Tendon of long digital extensor

Patellar ligament

Tibial tuberosity

Lateral   Medial

Figure 9–8.   Stifle joint of the dog.

The stifle joint has several ligaments of importance. There are six meniscal ligaments, two from each meniscus that attach to the tibia, one from the lateral meniscus to the femur, and an intermeniscal ligament that joins the two menisci. The cruciate ligaments join the femur to the tibia and lie within the joint cavity. The anterior (lateral) cruciate ligament runs from the medial aspect of the lateral femoral condyle to the cranial intercondylar area of the tibia. It inhibits cranial motion of the tibia in relation to the femur. The posterior (medial) cruciate ligament runs from the lateral aspect of the medial condyle of the femur caudally to the popliteal fossa of the caudal tibia. It prevents caudal movement of the tibia in relation to the femur. The tendon of insertion of the quadriceps femoris from the patella distally to its attachment on the tibial tuberosity is referred to as the patellar tendon. The infrapatellar fat pad lies between the fibrous and synovial layers of the joint capsule under the patellar ligament. The tendon of the long digital extensor originates on the lateral condyle of the femur and crosses the joint space on its craniolateral aspect.

The tarsal joint is a composite articulation like the carpal joint (Fig. 9–9). Only the tarsocrural joint will be discussed because there is little motion in the intertarsal and tarsometatarsal joints. The distal end of the fibula (lateral malleolus) can be felt as a small knob on the distolateral aspect of the crus. The medial part of the distal end of the tibia (medial malleolus) is a similarly raised area. These mark

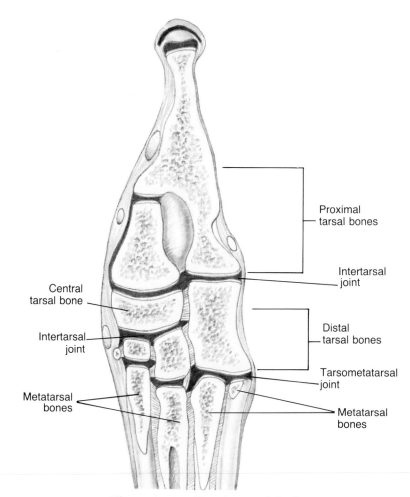

Proximal
tarsal bones

Intertarsal
joint

Central
tarsal bone

Distal
tarsal bones

Intertarsal
joint

Tarsometatarsal
joint

Metatarsal
bones

Metatarsal
bones

Figure 9–9. Tarsal joint of the dog.

the proximal extent of the tarsocrural joint. Distally, the ridges of
the trochlea of the talus can be felt with the joint extended. Lateral
to the trochlea is the calcaneus, which extends caudoproximally as
the tuber calcanei. The dorsal pedal artery crosses the joint space on
its craniomedial aspect.

Other Bony or Muscular Landmarks

The wings of the atlas are located caudal to the occipital area of the
skull and are directed in an almost dorsoventral manner. The transverse processes of cervical vertebrae two through five can be palpated on each side of the neck midway between the dorsal and
ventral aspects. The spinous processes of the fourth through the
thirteenth thoracic vertebrae are palpable on the dorsal midline
from just behind the scapulae. The eleventh thoracic vertebra is the
anticlinal vertebra, so named because its spinous process is perpendicular to the long axis of the spine while the spinous processes of
the vertebrae cranial to it are directed caudally and those caudal to it
are directed cranially. The spinous processes of the seven lumbar
vertebrae are all palpable along the dorsal midline. Caudolateral to
the seventh lumbar vertebra are the wings of the ilia, which protrude
dorsally in an arc directed from cranial to caudal. On either side of
the anus are the ischiatic tuberosities.

Observation

Note the animal's conformation, being aware of individual breed variations that are considered normal. Examine the posture of the standing animal. Does the animal have a wide- or narrow-based stance? Is there evidence of inward or outward deviation of the toes? Can you imagine a straight line being drawn from the point of the shoulder to the middle two toes or from the stifle to the middle two toes (Fig. 9–10)? Are the limbs symmetric in size and joint conformation? Is there evidence of muscle atrophy? Is the animal bearing weight symmetrically on all four limbs? Do the joints, especially the carpi and tarsi, appear to be in the normal weight-bearing position?

Poor conformation may predispose to abnormal stresses on bones and ligaments, resulting in lameness.

Decreased muscle mass is indicative of muscle atrophy, which can result from many causes such as nerve dysfunction or disuse.

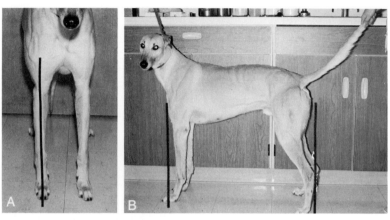

Figure 9–10. Normal conformation of a dog in a standing position is shown. *A*, Front view. *B*, Side view.

After observing the animal stand, ask the owner to walk the animal away from and toward you. Use an area that is free of obstruction and large enough to adequately assess the gait. Does the animal carry or drag any of the limbs? Is the animal bearing weight symmetrically on all limbs? Is there obvious movement of the head with the movement of the limbs? Lamenesses should be graded according to the scale in Table 9–2.

Ligament laxity secondary to metabolic disease such as hyperadrenocorticism or immune-mediated connective tissue disease such as rheumatoid arthritis may result in hyperextension of the carpus (Fig. 9–11).

Table 9–2 GRADES OF LAMENESS	
Grade	**Character**
I	Barely perceptible
II	Noticeable, but weight-bearing
III	Bears weight occasionally for balance
IV	Completely non–weight-bearing

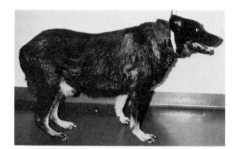

Figure 9–11. Severe ligament laxity is shown in a 12-year-old male shepherd cross with hyperadrenocorticism.

Dragging of the limb usually suggests neurologic disease as a cause of the lameness. Orthopedic lamenesses usually are characterized by holding the leg up off the ground if the lameness is severe enough.

"Head bobbing" is a useful indicator of the location of a lameness. The head is pulled up with the placement of the lame leg on the ground and moves down when the sound leg is placed on the ground.

In addition to obvious lamenesses, note any of the following: dragging of the toes, knuckling, shortened strides, toeing in or out, circumduction of a limb, hypermetria, trembling, ataxia, crossing over of the legs, and asymmetry of motion.

Have the owner trot the animal. This may accentuate minor lamenesses and aid in their diagnosis.

Circumduction of a foreleg may be indicative of the reluctance of the animal to flex the shoulder joint. Hypermetria, ataxia, knuckling, and crossing over suggest neurologic disease and will be discussed in Chapter 11. Shortened strides may be indicative of reluctance to extend the shoulder joint or more generalized pain.

Palpation

It is important to develop a routine for consistent and complete palpation of the musculoskeletal system. The order of the examination is not as important as the fact that items are not overlooked. It is not always necessary to complete a full orthopedic examination on all animals unless the chief complaint deals with this system or if the animal's problem is posing a diagnostic dilemma. Palpate and examine each leg from distal to proximal, flexing and extending the joints *individually* as you move up the leg. It is important to isolate the examination to specific parts. If a painful carpus is moved during the examination of the elbow joint, one may mistakenly conclude that the elbow is also painful. Palpate gently at first; if no pain is elicited and a problem is still suspected, more aggressive palpation is indicated. Be thorough; do not just examine the leg with a problem. Because of the bilateral symmetry of the musculoskeletal system normally, there is usually a good limb readily available for comparison.

Separate the toes and examine the skin between them. Are there areas of redness and/or swelling? Palpate the bones and joints of the feet, noting any pain, bony enlargements, or crepitus.

Degenerative arthritis, fractures, or luxations can give rise to crepitus when the joints are flexed or extended. Pain can be noted with infectious, traumatic, degenerative, or neoplastic processes. Painful bony swelling is most consistent with a bone tumor.

As you move proximally, flex and extend the carpus/tarsus (Figs. 9–12 and 9–13). Palpate the joint noting any effusion. Firmly palpate the bones of the crus and antebrachium (Fig. 9–14). Is there pain, swelling, crepitus, or heat noticed?

Effusion in the distal joints is consistent with idiopathic, non-erosive polyarthritis or other immune-mediated arthritis. Bone pain may be associated with panosteitis in the young dog or hypertrophic pulmonary osteoarthropathy in the older animal.

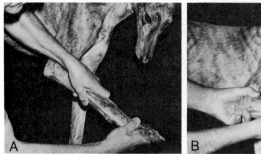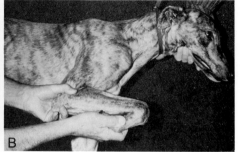

Figure 9–12. Normal range of motion of the canine carpus. *A*, Extension; *B*, flexion. (Courtesy of Dr. Donald Piermattei.)

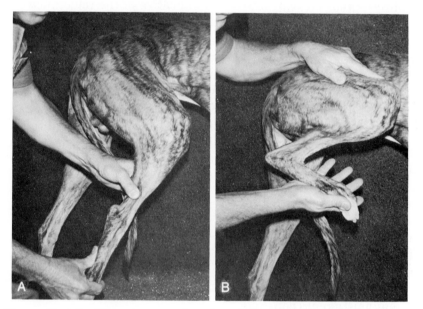

Figure 9–13. Normal range of motion of the canine tarsus. (Courtesy of Dr. Donald Piermattei.)

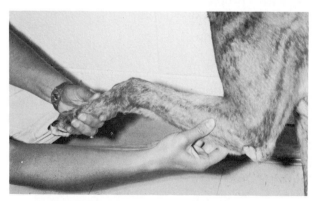

Figure 9–14. Palpation of the radius and ulna.

Flex and extend the elbow/stifle joint (Figs. 9–15 and 9–16). To assess the cruciate ligaments, place the thumb and forefinger of one hand on the lateral epicondyle of the femur and patella, respectively. With the other hand, place the thumb and forefinger on the head of the fibula and the proximal tibial crest, respectively. Gripping firmly with each hand, move the hands in opposite directions and note the amount of motion in the stifle (Fig. 9–17). Palpate the patella and, with the stifle extended, gently push the patella medially. Palpate the humerus/femur deeply.

A positive anterior drawer sign, movement of the tibia anteriorly in relation to the femur, is characteristic of a ruptured anterior cruciate ligament. Medial patellar luxation is commonly seen in toy breeds of dogs. The patella may be easily luxated by manipulation or may be permanently luxated depending on the severity.

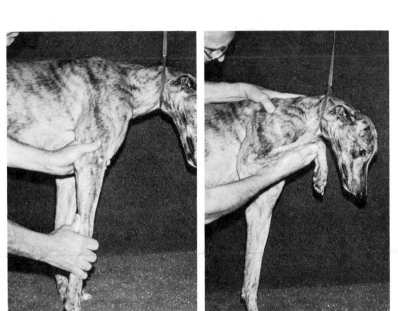

Figure 9–15. Normal range of motion of the canine elbow joint. (Courtesy of Dr. Donald Piermattei.)

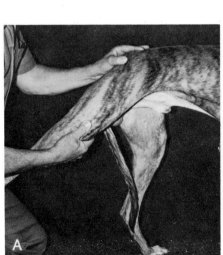
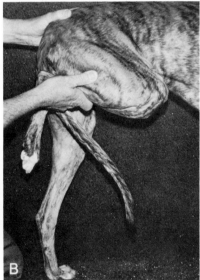

Figure 9–16. Normal range of motion of the canine stifle joint. (Courtesy of Dr. Donald Piermattei.)

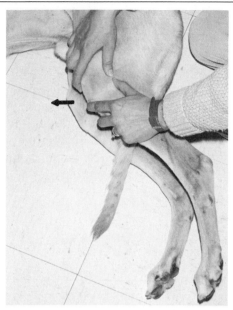

Figure 9–17. Technique for assessing cruciate ligament stability.

Move the shoulder/hip joints through their range of motion (Figs. 9–18 and 9–19). To assess the degree of laxity in the coxofemoral joint, place the animal in lateral recumbency with the leg to be examined up. Brace the animal with one hand over the lumbosacral area. With the other hand, hold the stifle and push dorsally as you abduct the limb (Fig. 9–21). Note any crepitus or sudden popping.

Crepitus upon movement of the coxofemoral joint suggests degenerative joint disease, fractures, or luxations. Luxations of the hip are most commonly in the antero-dorsal direction, which results in the affected limb being shorter than the normal limb. In addition, the limb is carried in an externally rotated position (Fig. 9–20).

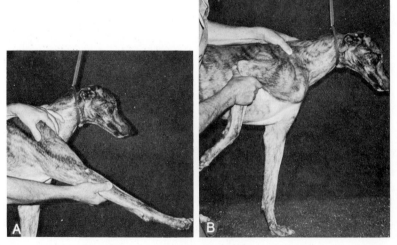

Figure 9–18. Normal range of motion of the canine shoulder joint. (Courtesy of Dr. Donald Piermattei.)

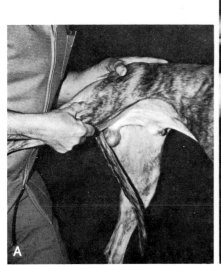

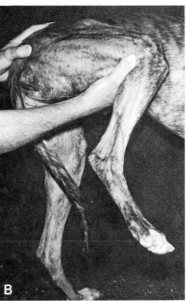

Figure 9–19. Normal range of motion of the canine coxofemoral joint. (Courtesy of Dr. Donald Piermattei.)

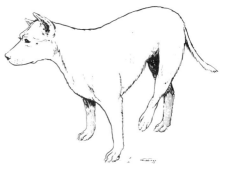

Figure 9–20. A dog that has a coxofemoral luxation. Note the external rotation of the stifle. (Used by permission. From Brinker WO, Piermattei DL, Flo GL: Handbook of Small Animal Orthopedics and Fracture Treatment, p 268. Philadelphia, WB Saunders, 1983.)

Hip dysplasia or coxofemoral joint laxity is indicated by a positive Ortolani sign (popping of the head of the femur back into the acetabulum when the femur is abducted) (Fig. 9–21).

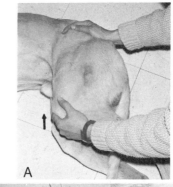

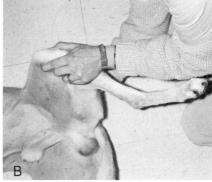

Figure 9–21. Assessment of coxofemoral joint laxity.

Palpate the scapula/ilium, noting pain, masses, or crepitus.

Gently dorsiflex and ventriflex the neck (Fig. 9–22). Move the head laterally in both directions, noting any pain, resistance, or asymmetry in the range of motion. Lateral flexion in most normal animals allows the nose to touch the lateral thorax. Palpate the spinous processes of the thoracic and lumbar vertebrae, pressing downward gently to note any pain. Are the muscles of the back and pelvic area symmetric? Palpate the tail for any pain, swelling, or crepitus.

Pain on manipulation of the neck suggests meningitis, cervical disc disease, trauma, or spinal neoplasia. Thoracolumbar disc disease, neoplasia, or infection may cause pain that is elicited by applying downward pressure on the dorsal spinous processes.

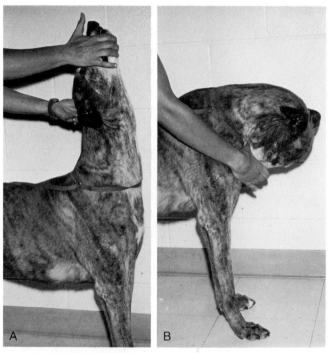

Figure 9–22. Normal range of motion of the cervical spine.

Auscultation and Percussion

Not useful in the examination of the musculoskeletal system.

DIFFERENCES IN THE CAT

Anatomically, there are some differences in the musculoskeletal system of the cat compared to the dog. Cats have a *suprahamate process* that projects caudally from the distal end of the spine of the scapula. The clavicle is well developed and osseous and can be palpated in some cats. There is a supracondylar foramen in the humerus through which the median nerve and brachial artery pass. The metatarsal bones are about twice as long as the metacarpal bones. Various muscles differ somewhat in their origin and/or insertion in the cat compared to the dog. This is of little significance in the physical examination.

Cats are often quite uncooperative and may be difficult to examine if a musculoskeletal problem is suspected. They are usually not trained to walk on a leash and thus frequently must be examined while walking freely around the examination room. Use of rigid restraint in the cat is usually counterproductive.

RECOMMENDED READING

1. Arnoczky SP, Tarvin GB: Physical Examination of the Musculoskeletal System. Vet Clin North Am 11(3):575, 1981.
2. Bates B: A Guide to Physical Examination and History Taking, 4th ed. Philadelphia, JB Lippincott, 1987.
3. Brinker WO, Piermattei DL, Flo GL: Handbook of Small Animal Orthopedics and Fracture Treatment. Philadelphia, WB Saunders, 1983.
4. Evans HB, Christensen GC: Miller's Anatomy of the Dog, 2nd ed. Philadelphia, WB Saunders, 1979.

Integumentary System

APPLIED ANATOMY

The skin is made up of the subcutis, dermis, and epidermis (Fig. 10–1). The subcutis contains fat and the blood and nerve supply to the skin. In addition, hair follicles and some glands are present in the subcutis. The dermis contains the hair follicles, sebaceous and sweat glands, blood vessels and lymphatics, and small branches of nerves. The epidermis is composed of the germinal layer of cells (stratum basale), the layer of daughter cells (stratum spinosum), the layer of cells with visible keratohyaline granules (stratum granulosum), the layer of fully cornified, non-nucleated cells (stratum luci-

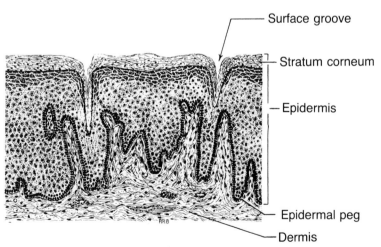

Figure 10–1. Basic histology of the skin. (Used by permission. From Evans HB, Christensen GC: Miller's Anatomy of the Dog, 2nd ed. Philadelphia, WB Saunders, 1979.)

dum), and the layer of fully cornified cells that are desquamating (stratum corneum). Not all of these layers are present in all areas of the skin. For instance, the stratum lucidum is found only in the foot pads of the dog and cat. The thickness of the epidermis varies over different parts of the body. It is very thick over the shoulder area where it is the most movable. The epidermis blends with the mucosa at mucocutaneous junctions.

The majority of the skin of the dog and cat is haired. The hair follicle (an inversion of the surface epidermis) is responsible for hair production. The outer and inner root sheaths are surrounded by a rich blood supply. Most of the hair follicles of dogs and cats are compound (Fig. 10–2). There are multiple hairs that emerge from the same follicular opening on the epidermal surface. These hairs share the same follicle down to the level of the sebaceous gland and then the follicle branches so that each hair has its own follicle and bulb. Usually, there is one primary or guard hair per follicle that is surrounded by multiple secondary or undercoat hairs. The follicles are usually in groups of three, arranged in irregular rows in the skin. The surface of the skin has scalelike folds from which the hairs emerge. The density of the follicles and the numbers and types of hairs within the follicle vary greatly with the breed of dog or cat.

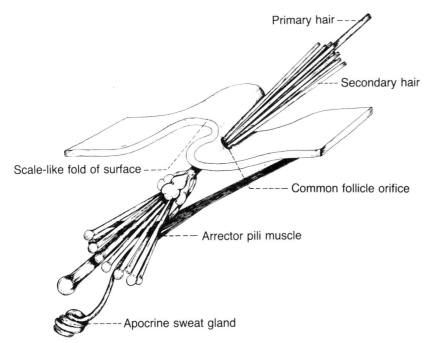

Figure 10–2. Structure of a compound hair follicle. (Used by permission. From Evans HB, Christensen GC: Miller's Anatomy of the Dog, 2nd ed. Philadelphia, WB Saunders, 1979.)

There are several specialized structures in the skin of dogs and cats. Specialized hairs include the tactile hairs of the muzzle and the eyelashes. The skin of the nose is usually heavily pigmented and thick. There are no glands present in its dermis or epidermis. The epidermis is marked by deep grooves that appear grossly as an irregular network of crevices. The skin of the foot pads is the thickest in the body. The surface of the pad is visibly roughened by projections of heavily keratinized epidermis. The pads are cushioned by subcutaneous fat and connective tissue. Merocrine sweat glands originate in this layer and travel through the dermis and epidermis to the surface. The skin of the scrotum is very thin and has few hair follicles. The tail gland area, on the dorsal aspect of the tail just distal to the tailhead, is an oval-shaped region of specialized skin. The hairs emerge singly from the follicles and the sebaceous glands are very extensive.

The claws are highly developed extensions of the skin over the third phalanx of each digit (Fig. 10–3). They are curved and flattened laterally. The epidermis is made of hardened, cornified cells that are fused to make a plate that is attached to the periosteum of the bone by the dermis. The dermis is well vascularized in this area.

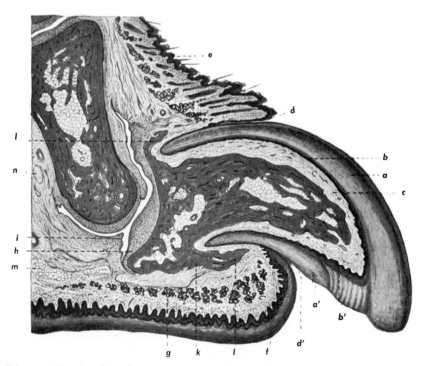

Figure 10–3. Complex structure of a claw. *a*, Stratum corneum of the epidermis of the claw: *a'*, stratum corneum of the epidermis of the sole. *b,b'*, Deep, noncornified epidermal layers of the dorsum and sole of the claw. *c*, Corium (papillated in the area of the sole). *d*, Claw fold. *d'*, Limiting furrow separating the sole from the digital pad. *e*, Skin with hair and glands. *f*, Epidermis of the digital pad with strata granulosum and lucidum. *g*, Tubular glands in the digital pad. *h*, Articular cartilage of the third phalanx. *i*, Meniscus. *k*, Sharpey fibers from a tendon insertion. *l*, Ungual crest. *m*, Fat cushion with the digital pad. *n*, Lamellar corpuscle. (Used by permission. From Trautmann A, Fiebiger J: Fundamentals of the Histology of Domestic Animals. Ithaca, NY, Cornell University Press, 1952.)

The anal sac is a reservoir for the secretions of the anal glands. There are two sacs, located ventrolateral to the anus between the external and internal anal sphincter (Fig. 10–4). The openings of the sacs are present in the cutaneous area on each side of the anus just below a horizontal line that bisects the anus.

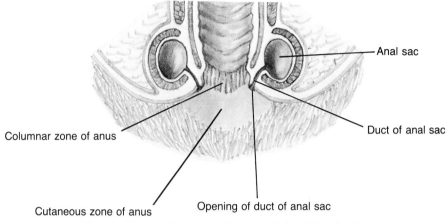

Columnar zone of anus

Anal sac

Duct of anal sac

Cutaneous zone of anus

Opening of duct of anal sac

Figure 10–4. Location of the anal glands in the dog.

The mammary glands are modified cutaneous glands that are arranged in two bilaterally symmetric rows on either side of the midline. They number 8 to 12 depending on the size of the animal. Males have rudimentary glands; however, the mammary glands of females undergo obvious changes during pregnancy and lactation. The glandular tissue secretes milk into the gland sinus. From there the milk flows into the teat sinus, into the teat canal, and out the teat orifices, which are multiple in the dog.

The color of normal skin varies with the breed of dog or cat. It is dependent on the number of melanocytes in the skin as well as the number, size, and disposition of melanin granules within the melanocytes. The skin is usually pale tan in color but may have patches of gray to black or may be entirely gray.

Observation

From a distance, look the animal over, noting the haircoat. Is it shiny and well-groomed? Does the animal appear to be in good health? Note the general body condition. If there is a skin problem, is it generalized or localized? The distribution of the lesions should be noted. Are they symmetrically or asymmetrically distributed?

Be as systematic as possible in the evaluation of the skin and coat. Start with the dorsal surface and then observe the lateral surfaces. Roll the animal on its back to observe the ventrum.

Be sure to have adequate lighting when examining the skin. If necessary, utilize a separate light source and a magnifying lens or loupe to better visualize lesions.

Run your hands against the grain of the hair and visualize the skin underneath. Is the haircoat thin (hypotrichosis) or absent (alopecia) in places? Does the skin appear red or inflamed? Are there any primary lesions present (Table 10–1)? Are there any secondary lesions (Table 10–2)? Is there any particular arrangement of the lesions? Do you see any external parasites? Is the skin or hair discolored in any way?

Many underlying metabolic diseases such as hyperadrenocorticism and hypothyroidism affect the skin as well as other organ systems. Clues to the etiology of a skin problem may, therefore, lie in the careful inspection of the whole animal. Obesity is a common complaint of owners with hypothyroid animals and may also be seen with hyperadrenocorticism.

A generalized skin problem may imply chronicity, increased severity, or underlying metabolic disorder leading to immunocompromise. An example of a localized skin disease is discoid lupus erythematosus (Fig. 10–5).

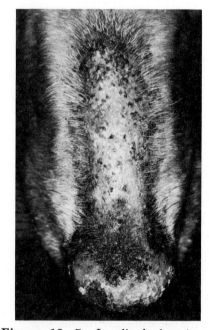

Figure 10–5. Localized alopecia on the bridge of the nose in a dog with discoid lupus erythematosus. (Courtesy of Dr. Stephen White, Colorado State University.)

Many skin disorders have typical patterns of hair loss or skin lesions that can be a significant

Table 10–1 PRIMARY SKIN LESIONS	
Lesion Type	**Description**
Macule	Circumscribed spot that is flattened; <1 cm in diameter; color change noted
Papule	Circumscribed, solid, raised area; <1 cm in diameter; usually pink or red in color
Nodule	Circumscribed, solid, raised area; >1 cm in diameter; extends into deeper layers of the skin
Tumor	Neoplastic mass that may involve the skin and subcutaneous tissue
Pustule	Circumscribed area filled with pus; intraepidermal or follicular in location; yellow or red in color
Wheal	Circumscribed raised area that appears and disappears in a short period of time; white-pink in color
Vesicle	Circumscribed raised area filled with clear fluid

Table 10–2
SECONDARY SKIN LESIONS

Lesion Type	Description
Scale	Loose clumps of cornified cell layer
Crust	Dried accumulation of exudate on the surface of a lesion; aggregation of pus, blood, scale, and hair
Scar	Fibrous tissue that is a result of healing of a lesion; dermis and subcutis involved
Ulcer	Interruption of the epidermis leaving the dermis exposed; thickened epidermis around the periphery
Excoriation	Superficial loss of areas of epidermis caused by self-trauma
Lichenification	An area of skin that is thickened and hard; often hyperpigmented
Abnormal pigmentation	Change in skin color; usually related to melanin deposition, but other colors are possible
Comedone	Hair follicle plugged with cells, dirt, oil, and debris
Hyperkeratosis	Increased thickness of the cornified layer of the epidermis
Fissure	Linear cracks in the epidermis and/or dermis

diagnostic aid. A dermatology text should be consulted for specifics of various diseases.

Bilaterally symmetric alopecia is suggestive of an endocrine cause of the dermatologic problem (Fig. 10–6).

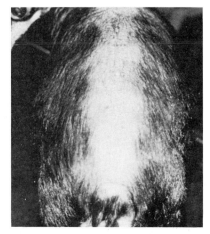

Figure 10–6. Endocrine alopecia typically has a symmetric pattern of hair loss.

Seborrhea can be characterized by excessive flakiness to the skin and is a result of increased scale formation and abnormal sebum production.

Primary skin lesions are the result of the underlying disorder and may support an etiologic diagnosis. Secondary lesions, on the other hand, result from trauma, infection, or progression of the primary disease. They are usually not helpful in the diagnosis of the problem.

Flea-bite dermatitis has a characteristic distribution of lesions over the tailhead region. Fleas may be seen moving through the thinned hair.

Increased melanin deposition, or hyperpigmentation, is often a sign of chronic dermatitis. It can also be indicative of endocrine dermatopathies such as hyperadrenocorticism (Fig. 10–7). Loss of skin pigment (leukoderma) or hair pigment (leukotrichia) can be congenital or acquired as a result of trauma, infections, or radiation. Hypopigmentation can be idiopathic.

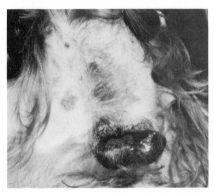

Figure 10–7. Hyperpigmentation, an increase in the amount of melanin in the skin, in a dog with hyperadrenocorticism.

Examine the feet carefully by lifting each one and spreading the toes apart. Look at both the dorsal and ventral surfaces for redness, swelling, exudation, or cracking. Are the toenails broken, cracked, or brittle?

Pododermatitis can have a number of etiologies; however, the feet appear swollen and red, and may crack and ooze serum regardless of the cause (Fig. 10–8).

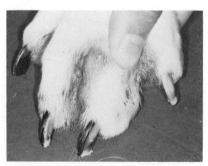

Figure 10–8. Pododermatitis has a variety of etiologies.(Courtesy of Dr. Stephen White, Colorado State University.)

Examine the mucocutaneous junctions, noting any ulceration, petechia, or bulla formation.

Autoimmune skin diseases may affect the mucocutaneous junctions along with the feet, nose, and other areas of the skin (Fig. 10–9).

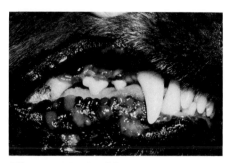

Figure 10–9. Mucocutaneous junctions may be a site of involvement with the immune-mediated skin diseases such as pemphigus vulgaris.

Palpation

Feel the haircoat for abnormalities in texture and for excessive dryness or oiliness. As you pass your hands over the animal's body, note any masses or swellings in the skin. Are any areas painful as they are palpated? Does the animal react adversely to separating and examining the toes? Note the thickness of the skin as well as its elasticity and distensibility. Does the hair epilate or fall out easily?

Excessive oiliness to the coat in addition to excessive scaliness is consistent with seborrhea oleosa.

Skin tumors account for approximately one third of the tumors diagnosed in dogs. The ability to differentiate benign from malignant lesions begins with the physical examination. Benign lesions tend to be slow-growing and well-encapsulated and may be pedunculated.

Painful lumps may be indicative of abscessation.

The skin is often thinner than normal in many endocrine dermatopathies.

Palpate the mammary chains, noting any masses or discharge (Fig. 10–10).

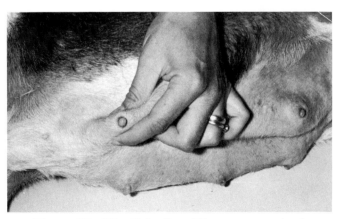

Figure 10–10. Palpation of the mammary gland.

Mammary neoplasia may vary in presentation from a small, firm, pea-sized lump to diffuse erythematous thickening of the skin. Mastitis is most commonly seen 1 to 3 weeks post partum and is associated with hot, swollen, painful glands from which discolored milk can be expressed.

Examine the anal glands using a gloved index finger inside the rectum and the thumb externally.

Impactions of the anal sacs feel like hard, acorn-sized nodules that are difficult at best to express. Infection of the anal sacs results in purulent exudate within the gland. Anal sac abscesses may rupture through the skin of the perineum lateral to the anus.

Describe any lesions by their distribution, pattern or arrangement, location within the skin, consistency, quality, and color.

The indolent ulcer or rodent ulcer is a thickened, ulcerated area on the rostral aspect of the upper lip (Fig. 10–11).

Percussion and Auscultation

Not useful in the examination of the skin.

DIFFERENCES IN THE CAT

The cat's skin is thinner than the dog's in general. The foot pads are normally smooth in the cat. Secondary hair follicles are arranged in groups of two, three, four, or five around a primary hair follicle. In addition to tactile hairs of the muzzle and eyebrows, cats have tylotrich hairs scattered throughout their haircoat. These hairs emerge singly from a large hair follicle and are thought to be rapid-adapting mechanoreceptors.

The eosinophilic granuloma complex is an idiopathic skin disease of cats. It has several presentations including the indolent ulcer (Fig. 10–11), eosinophilic plaque, and linear granuloma.

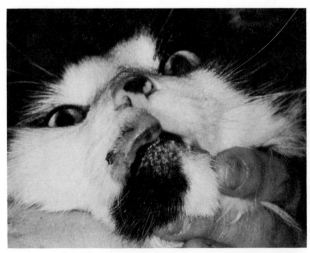

Figure 10–11. An indolent (rodent) ulcer on the upper lip of a cat. (Courtesy of Dr. Stephen White, Colorado State University.)

RECOMMENDED READING

1. Evans HB, Christensen GC: Miller's Anatomy of the Dog, 2nd ed. Philadelphia, WB Saunders, 1979.
2. Muller GH, Kirk RW, Scott DW: Small Animal Dermatology, 3rd ed. Philadelphia, WB Saunders, 1983.

Nervous System

APPLIED ANATOMY

The Brain

The brain consists of three structures — the cerebrum, the subcortical area, and the cerebellum (Fig. 11–1). The cerebrum is divided into two hemispheres, each of which has four lobes — the frontal, parietal, occipital, and temporal. The subcortical structures consist of the basal nuclei, thalamus, hypothalamus, midbrain, pons, and medulla oblongata. The latter five structures are also referred to as the brain stem. Most of the cranial nerves arise from this area of the brain. The cerebellum is caudal to the cerebrum and separated from it by the osseous tentorium.

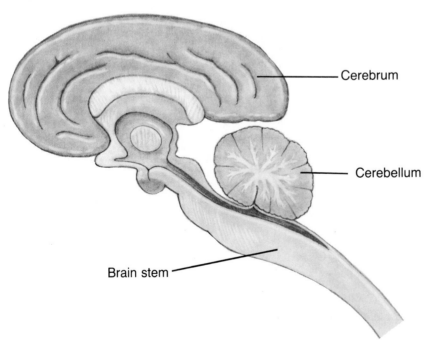

Cerebrum

Cerebellum

Brain stem

Figure 11–1. Gross anatomy of the canine brain showing the cerebrum, cerebellum, and brain stem.

The Spinal Cord

The spinal cord is a cylindric mass of nervous tissue that continues from the brain stem. It is housed within the bony vertebral column and ends at the level of the fifth or sixth lumbar vertebra in the dog. Ascending and descending tracts connect the neurons of the spinal cord with the cerebrum and cerebellum. The spinal cord is divided into 36 segments, corresponding to areas where nerve fibers enter and exit the cord for the paired spinal nerves. Each spinal nerve is formed by the convergence of a dorsal (sensory) root and a ventral (motor) root (Fig. 11–2). There are eight cervical, thirteen thoracic, seven lumbar, three sacral, and five coccygeal cord segments. The spinal cord has a central core of gray matter, the nerve cell bodies, which is surrounded by white matter, the nerve fiber tracts. The nerve cell bodies within the gray matter are predominantly motor neurons or interneurons. The sensory nerve cell bodies are located outside the spinal cord in the dorsal root ganglia.

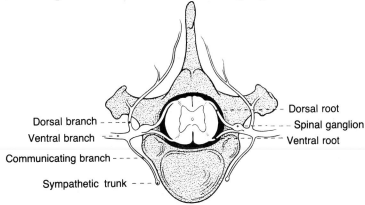

Figure 11–2. Spinal nerves are composed of the dorsal and ventral nerve roots. (Used by permission. From Evans HB, Christensen GC: Miller's Anatomy of the Dog, 2nd ed, p 573. Philadelphia, WB Saunders, 1979.)

A Reflex Arc

A reflex is an involuntary reaction to a defined stimulus. In most cases, elicitation of a reflex tests only the cord segments involved in that reflex. There are three components of a reflex arc (Fig. 11–3).

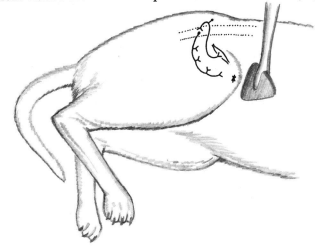

Figure 11–3. A reflex arc has afferent and efferent nerves and an effector muscle.

The first is the afferent or sensory component, which carries information from the periphery *to* the spinal cord. Usually, with the tendon (myotatic) reflexes, the stimulus is stretching of a receptor apparatus within the tendon that is tapped with a pleximeter. Within the spinal cord, the afferent nerve fiber synapses with the motor nerve cell body and the impulse travels to the effector organ, the muscle, which responds by contraction.

The Motor Pathways

The motor pathways are those tracts that carry information to the lower motor neurons from higher centers. These include the corticospinal, rubrospinal, reticulospinal, vestibulospinal, and tectospinal tracts and the medial longitudinal fasciculus. The location of these tracts is shown in Figure 11–4.

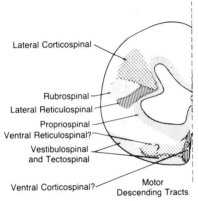

Figure 11–4. Location of the motor tracts within the spinal cord. (Used by permission. From Hoerlein BF: Canine Neurology, 3rd ed. Philadelphia, WB Saunders, 1978.)

The Sensory Pathways

The sensory pathways carry information *from* the periphery to the central nervous system. The fasciculi cuneatus and gracilis, spinothalamic, spinocerebellar, and spinotectal tracts perform this function. Their location within the spinal cord is shown in Figure 11–5.

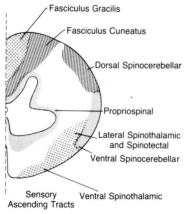

Figure 11–5. Location of the sensory pathways within the spinal cord. (Used by permission. From Hoerlein BF: Canine Neurology, 3rd ed. Philadelphia, WB Saunders, 1978.)

A sensory map of the dog is depicted in Figure 11–6. This relates the location of a sensory deficit to a corresponding spinal nerve and cord segment.

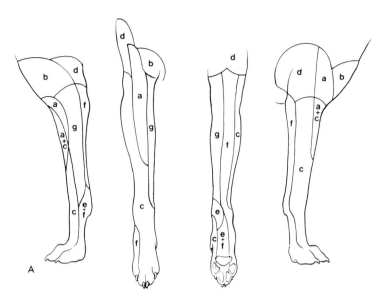

A

a, Axillary nerve (C6,7,8)

b, Branchiocephalic nerve (C5,6)

c, Radial nerve (C7,8,T1,2)

d, Thoracic nerve (T2-T4)

e, Median nerve (includes the branch from the musculocutaneous nerve) (C6,7,8,T1,2)

f, Ulnar nerve (C8,T1,2)

g, Musclocutaneous nerve (C6,7,8)

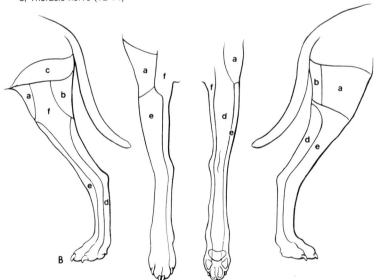

B

a, Lateral cutaneous femoral nerve (L3,4,5)

b, Caudal cutaneous femoralnerve (L7-S1,2)

c, Genitofemoral nerve (L3,4)

d, Tibial nerve (L6,7,S1)

e, Peroneal nerve (L6,7,S1)

f, Saphenous nerve (femoral) (L4,5)

Figure 11–6. Sensory map of the dog. *A*, Right thoracic limb of the dog. *B*, Right pelvic limb of the dog. (Used by permission. From Oliver JE, Lorenz MD: Handbook of Veterinary Neurologic Diagnosis, pp 53, 54. Philadelphia, WB Saunders, 1983.)

The Cranial Nerves

Table 11–1 summarizes the cranial nerves, their origin, and their function.

Table 11–1 THE CRANIAL NERVES			
Number	**Name**	**Origin**	**Function**
I	Olfactory	Olfactory bulb	Sense of smell
II	Optic	Optic chiasm	Vision
III	Oculomotor	Midbrain	Pupillary constriction, elevation of the upper eyelid, most of the ocular movements
IV	Trochlear	Midbrain	Motor to dorsal oblique muscle of the eye
V	Trigeminal	Pons	Sensation of the face and eye, motor to muscles of mastication
VI	Abducens	Pons	Motor to retractor bulbi and lateral rectus muscles of the eye
VII	Facial	Pons	Motor to the facial muscles, sensory to the anterior two thirds of the tongue
VIII	Acoustic	Medulla	Senses of hearing and balance
IX	Glossopharyngeal	Medulla	Sensory to the root of the tongue, pharynx, middle ear; motor to the muscles of the pharynx
X	Vagus	Medulla	Motor and sensory to the larynx, pharynx, soft palate; parasympathetic innervation of organs in the abdomen and chest
XI	Accessory	Medulla	Motor to the trapezius, sternocephalicus, and brachiocephalicus muscles
XII	Hypoglossal	Medulla	Motor to the tongue muscles

The Pupillary Light Response

The pupillary light response is dependent on the function of the oculomotor nerve, the optic nerve, sympathetic pathways, and the integrative centers in the midbrain. When a light source is focused on the retina, the normal iris constricts. This is called the *direct response.* The *consensual* or *indirect response* is constriction of the contralateral pupil as well. When the light is withdrawn, the pupils gradually relax and dilate.

Techniques of Examination   Abnormalities

The appropriate extent of a neurologic examination varies from patient to patient. Guidelines for a general screening of the nervous system are provided in this chapter. Further testing may be necessary to better define abnormalities. A textbook of veterinary neurology should then be consulted.

Observation

Note the animal's gait, posture, and mental status from a distance. Is the animal aware of its surroundings and responsive to external stimuli? Is the animal able to walk?

Examination of the cranial nerves is outlined in Table 11–2.

Dogs that are mentally dull or exhibit compulsive behavior such as circling or head pressing may have neurologic disorders caused by intra- or extracranial abnormalities.

Table 11–2
EXAMINATION OF THE CRANIAL NERVES

Nerve	Test	Response NORMAL	ABNORMAL
I. Olfactory	Volatile substance	Sniff, recoil, nose lick	No response
II. Optic	Menace	Blink	No blink
	Pupillary light reflex	Direct, consensual responses present	No direct or consensual responses
III. Oculomotor	Pupillary light reflex	Direct, consensual responses present	No direct response, consensual intact
	Observe eye follow an object	Normal eye movement	Impaired ocular movement in ventral, dorsal, and medial directions
IV. Trochlear	Observe	Normal eye position	Dorsomedial strabismus
V. Trigeminal	Observe	Can close jaw	Jaw drop
	Palpate temporalis	Normal muscle tone	Muscle atrophy
	Corneal reflex	Eye blink	No blink
	Palpebral reflex	Eye blink	No blink
VI. Abducens	Observe	Normal eye position	Medial strabismus
VII. Facial	Observe	Facial symmetry	Lip droop
	Corneal reflex	Eye blink	No blink
	Palpebral reflex	Eye blink	No blink
	Menace	Eye blink	No blink
VIII. Acoustic	Handclap	Startle response	No response
	Move head horizontally, vertically	Normal nystagmus	No response, resting or positional nystagmus
	Observe	Normal head posture	Head tilt
	Righting response	Normal righting	Unable to right
IX. Glossopharyngeal	Gag reflex	Swallow	No response
X. Vagus	Gag reflex	Swallow	No response
	Oculocardiac reflex	Bradycardia	No response
	Laryngeal reflex	Cough	No response
XI. Accessory	Palpate neck muscles	Normal muscle tone	Muscle atrophy
XII. Hypoglossal	Tongue stretch	Retraction of tongue	No response

Postural Reactions

The postural reactions include wheelbarrowing, hemistanding, hemiwalking, hopping, and placing responses. These tests evaluate the ascending and descending pathways in the spinal cord, higher brain centers, touch/pressure receptors in the skin, and stretch receptors in muscles, tendons, and joints. The main value of these tests is to detect subtle defects that are manifest by asymmetry in the response of each side.

Wheelbarrowing. Figure 11–7 shows the technique of wheelbarrowing, in which the animal is forced to walk on only the front limbs while the rear limbs are held in the air. Normal animals move the forelimbs in a symmetric, alternating pattern with the head extended.

An asymmetric movement of the front limbs when wheelbarrowing indicates that the lesion involves the cervical spinal cord or the nerves originating from it.

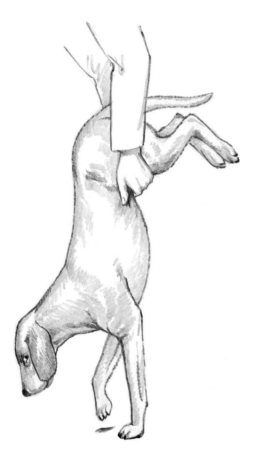

Figure 11–7. Wheelbarrowing.

Hemiwalking and Hemistanding. Hold the front and rear limbs on one side of the animal's body up off the ground (Fig. 11–8). Next force the animal to move forward or laterally. A normal animal will try to maintain the limbs in a vertical position under the body. There should be symmetry between the right and left sides of the animal.

Exaggerated or hypermetric responses to hemiwalking are consistent with cerebellar disease.

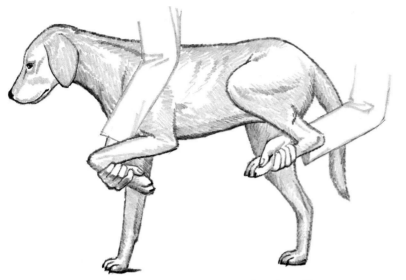

Figure 11–8.   Hemiwalking/hemistanding.

An asymmetric response in any of the four limbs helps to localize the source of the neurologic problem.

Hopping.   The hopping response is elicited by holding all of the animal's legs off the ground except for one (Fig. 11–9). The animal is then moved forward, backward, and laterally. The normal animal will respond by moving its leg in the direction of the movement in a hopping fashion in an attempt to keep the leg under the body for support.

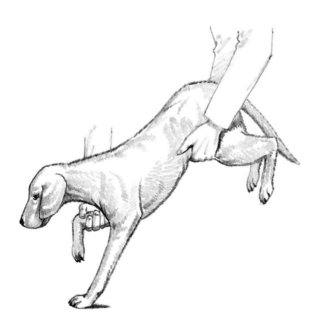

Figure 11–9.   Hopping.

Proprioception.   Test conscious proprioception in all four legs by gently flexing the metacarpal (-tarsal) -phalangeal joints and plac-

Patients with peripheral nerve dysfunction or spinal cord lesions may have a loss of proprioception as indicated by a failure to right the paw within 1 to 3 seconds.

ing the dorsal surface of the paw on the floor (Fig. 11–10). Repeat this several times per leg to get an accurate assessment of this function.

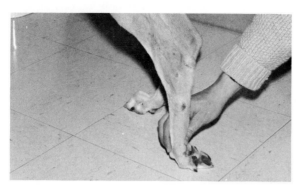

Figure 11–10.   To assess proprioception, place the animal's paw on the floor with the knuckles down and note the time it takes for the animal to right its paw.

Spinal Cord Reflexes

With a pleximeter, test the tendon or myotatic reflexes.

Patellar Reflex.   Place the animal in lateral recumbency with the limb to be examined in the up position. Allow the animal to relax. With the limb in the relaxed state, gently tap the patellar tendon at its middle with the broad base of the pleximeter (Fig. 11–11). The normal response is a quick extension of the stifle joint.

Absence of a response can be seen with a fracture of the femur without specific neurologic damage.

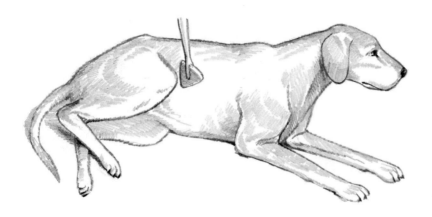

Figure 11–11.   Patellar reflex.

Gastrocnemius Reflex. With the animal in the same position, sharply tap the gastrocnemius tendon with the pleximeter (Fig. 11–12). The normal response is slight extension followed by flexion of the hock.

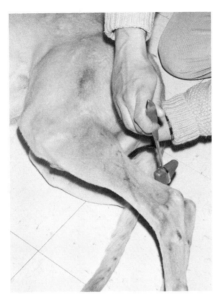

Figure 11–12. Gastrocnemius reflex.

Triceps Reflex. With the animal in the same position as above, tap the tendon of insertion of the triceps just proximal to the olecranon (Fig. 11–13). The normal response is slight extension of the elbow.

The forelimb reflexes may be difficult to see in normal animals, but contraction may be felt if the muscle is palpated when trying to elicit the reflex.

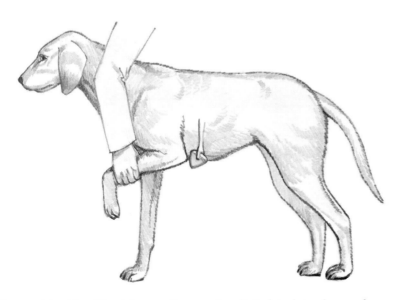

Figure 11–13. The triceps reflex can be elicited in lateral recumbency or standing as pictured.

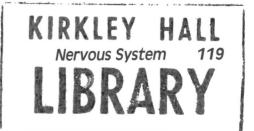

Flexor Response. The flexor responses can be tested in the front and rear limbs by gently compressing the foot pads to elicit a painful stimulus. The normal response is withdrawal of the limb (Fig. 11–14). Extension of the opposite rear leg when the contralateral toes are pinched is termed the crossed extensor reflex.

The *crossed extensor reflex* is elicited when there has been damage to the spinal cord above the segments being tested. It is characterized by extension of the leg opposite the leg to which a painful stimulus is being applied.

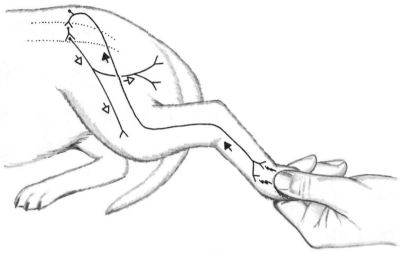

Figure 11–14. Flexor response.

Panniculus Reflex. The panniculus reflex is elicited by touching the skin over the back on either side of the vertebral column with a sharp object or pinching the skin gently with hemostat forceps. The normal response is contraction of the subcutaneous muscles at the point of stimulation.

Loss of the *panniculus reflex* helps to localize a neurologic problem. The lesion is one intervertebral space caudal to the level at which the first response is elicited, when stimulating from a caudal to a cranial direction.

Anal Reflex. Gentle tactile stimulation of the perineal region should elicit the anal reflex. Contraction of the external anal sphincter normally results.

Grading of Reflexes

It is useful in the localization of the neurologic deficit to grade the reflexes according to the following guidelines.

Grade	Description
0	No response
1	Hyporeflexia (less than normal response)
2	Normal response
3	Hyperreflexia (greater than normal response)
4	Clonus (repetitive response)

Reflexes that are graded 3 or 4 are consistent with *an upper motor neuron lesion.* Damage to the spinal cord above the segment where the nerves to the affected limb emerge results in a loss of the inhibitory neuron modulating effect on the reflexes. Grade 0 or 1 reflexes are considered to be a result of damage to the peripheral nerves or spinal cord at the segment where the nerves to the affected limb emerge. This is referred to as *a lower motor neuron lesion.*

Sensory Evaluation

Except for conscious proprioception, sensory evaluation is usually limited to tests of the perception of pain. *Superficial pain* is tested by gently squeezing the foot pads and watching for a pain response in the animal. These responses may be vocalization, dilation of the pupil, or moving the head to the side of the stimulus. Withdrawal of the limb is a segmental reflex and therefore cannot be used to assess pain perception. *Deep pain* is tested by squeezing the toes firmly. The same responses as above should be noted. Pricking the skin over various regions of the body, legs, and face may be done to map a sensory deficit.

Functional Relationships

Because of the location of the tracts within the spinal cord, there is a fairly consistent order in which functions are lost when the spinal cord is damaged. The initial function to be diminished is conscious proprioception, followed by superficial pain. Voluntary motor activity is lost as the trauma worsens. Deep pain is the last response to disappear and indicates severe spinal cord damage. In general, as more of these four functions are lost, both the damage and the prognosis for recovery worsen.

Palpation

Palpate the muscles during the examination of the animal for assessment of tone. Note any atrophy or lack of tone to the muscles.

Neurogenic muscular atrophy is rapid in onset and dramatic. In addition to cervical spine disease, neck pain can be associated with atlantoaxial subluxation or atlanto-occipital dysplasia.

Dorsiflex and ventriflex the cervical spine, noting any pain or resistance (see Fig. 9–22).

Palpate the spine, noting the symmetry of the vertebral column as well as the epaxial musculature. Gently apply downward pressure on each of the dorsal spinous processes of the thoracolumbar vertebrae. Is there evidence of pain?

Pain elicited by palpation of the vertebra is indicative of thoraco-lumbar disc disease, neoplasia, or discospondylitis.

Palpate high in the axillary space, noting any masses or pain (Fig. 11–15).

Pain in the axillary space may be indicative of a brachial plexus neurofibroma.

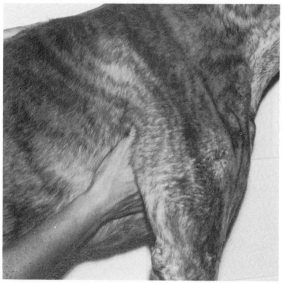

Figure 11–15. Palpation of the axillary space.

During the rectal examination, palpate and apply pressure dorsally to the lumbosacral area in the dog. Note any pain response.

Lumbosacral instability is often associated with pain elicited by upward pressure on the lumbosacral junction during a rectal examination.

Auscultation and Percussion

Not useful in the examination of the nervous system.

DIFFERENCES IN THE CAT

The cat is much more difficult to examine neurologically than the dog because of its uncooperative nature. The lack of an expected response may not be due to a neurologic deficit but simply the cat's refusal to respond.

RECOMMENDED READING

1. Averill DR: The neurologic examination. Vet Clin North Am 11(3):511, 1981.
2. Bailey CS, Kitchell RL: Clinical evaluation of the cutaneous innervation of the canine thoracic limb. J Am Anim Hosp Assoc 20:939, 1984.
3. Evans HB, Christensen GC: Miller's Anatomy of the Dog, 2nd ed. Philadelphia, WB Saunders, 1979.
4. Hoerlein BF: Canine Neurology, Diagnosis and Treatment, 3rd ed. Philadelphia, WB Saunders, 1978.
5. Oliver JE, Lorenz MD: Handbook of Veterinary Neurologic Diagnosis. Philadelphia, WB Saunders, 1983.

Lymphatic System

APPLIED ANATOMY

Only the superficial lymph nodes will be discussed here as they pertain to the physical examination. In addition, the spleen will be discussed in this section.

Lymph nodes are the functional units of the lymphoid system. They have a well-defined structure including a cortex and medulla and are surrounded by a fibrous capsule. In addition to providing an environment for lymphocyte production, they provide a storehouse for lymphocytes and a filtration system for blood. Lymph nodes are located in places that do not interfere with the function of other organ systems and yet are somewhat protected. Commonly, they are embedded in subcutaneous fat on the flexor (Fig. 12–1) surfaces of joints.

The lymph nodes of importance in the dog and cat are the mandibular, prescapular (both of which have been discussed in Chapter 4), axillary, inguinal, sublumbar (discussed in Chapter 7), and popliteal lymph nodes. Figure 12-1 illustrates the locations of these nodes.

Lymphatic vessels carry tissue fluid, foreign particles, and lymphocytes to (afferent) and from (efferent) the lymph node. With some exceptions, lymphatics parallel veins in their course through the body. They provide a means of returning fluid and cells lost from the veins and arteries to the systemic circulation.

The tonsils have already been described in Chapter 4.

The spleen parallels the greater curvature of the stomach and therefore lies in the left anterior quadrant of the abdomen. The shape of the spleen is irregular, but in general it is a flattened organ that is longer than it is wide. The dorsal extremity of the spleen lies among the diaphragm, the left kidney, and the fundus of the stomach. It is

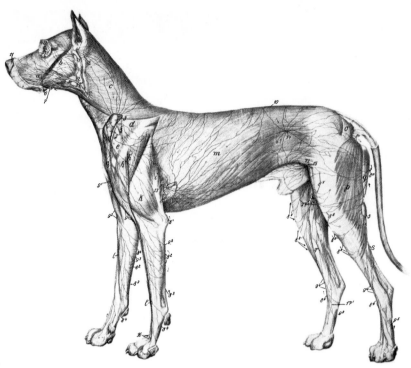

1, Parotid lymph node
2, 2', 2'', Mandibular lymph nodes
3, 3', Superficial cervical lymph nodes
4, Accessory axillary lymph node
5, Popliteal lymph node
6, Lymph vessels of the gums on
   the buccal side of the maxillary teeth
7, Lymph vessels of the gums on
   the buccal side of the mandibular teeth
8¹ to 8⁸, Lymph vessels which course to
   the medial side of the limb
   (those numbered 8⁵ to 8⁸ go to the
   superficial inguinal lymph nodes)
9¹, Lymph vessels of the skin of
   the cranial pectoral region
9² to 9⁵, Lymph vessels which course to
   the lateral side of the limb
10, Lymph vessel which crosses over
   the dorsal midline
11, Lymph vessels of the muzzle
12, Lymph vessel which passes deep to
   the medial retropharyngeal lymph node
13, 13', Lymph vessels which go to
   the axillary lymph node
14, Lymph vessels which go to
   the medial iliac lymph node

15, Lymph vessels which enter the
   superficial inguinal lymph nodes
16, Lymph vessels which pass from the
   palmar to the dorsal side of the forepaw
17, 17', Lymph vessels which go to
   the superficial inguinal lymph nodes
   a, Cheek muscles
   b, Masseter muscle
   c, c', Platysma and sphincter colli muscle
   d, M. trapezius cervicalis
   e, M. omotransversarius
   f, M. supraspinatus
   g, M. brachiocephalicus
   h, h', M. deltoideus
   i, k, Long and lateal head of the M. triceps brachii
   l, Antebrachial cephalic vein
   l', Accessory cephalic vein
   m, M. cutaneus trunci
   n, Fold of the flank
   o, M. gluteus superficialis
   p, M. biceps femoris
   q, M. semitendinosus
   r, Medial saphenous vein
   s, Lateral saphenous vein
   t, Medial femoral lymph node
   u, v, Upper and lower eyelid

Figure 12–1. Peripheral lymph nodes of importance. (Used by permission. From Evans HB, Christensen GC: Miller's Anatomy of the Dog, 2nd ed. Philadelphia, WB Saunders, 1979.)

relatively fixed in position by the gastrosplenic ligament, a portion of the omentum that attaches the spleen to the stomach. The ventral extremity is more freely movable. When the spleen is contracted, the entire spleen is tucked up under the ribs. With splenic enlargement, the ventral extremity moves caudoventrally. The tip of the spleen may cross the midline on the ventral floor of the abdomen.

Observation

Note any visible enlargement of superficial lymph nodes.

Visible enlargement of the superficial lymph nodes is most often associated with neoplasia or infectious inflammation (Fig. 12–5).

Note the presence of localized or generalized edema.

Local compromise of lymphatic drainage results in edema.

Palpation

Palpate each of the superficial lymph nodes (Figs. 12-2 to 12-4). The texture as well as the size and shape is important. Note any pain associated with palpation. If enlargement is present, is it symmetric or not?

Firm lymph nodes are consistent with neoplasia or inflammation. Necrosis may cause the lymph nodes to be softer than normal.

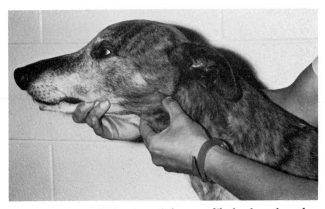

Figure 12–2. Palpation of the mandibular lymph node.

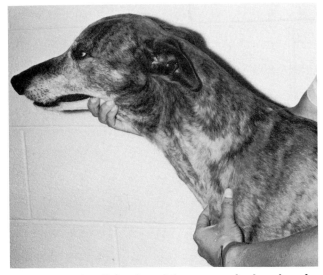

Figure 12–3. Palpation of the prescapular lymph node.

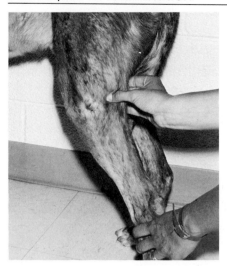

Figure 12–4. Palpation of the popliteal lymph node.

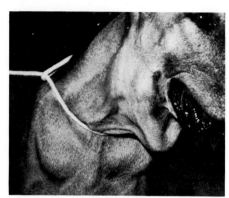

Figure 12–5. Enlarged peripheral lymph node in a dog with lymphosarcoma. (Courtesy of Dr. Joyce Obradovich, Colorado State University.)

Palpate the cranial ventral portion of the abdomen for the spleen. Its elongated shape and sharp edges make it easy to identify unless it is under the costal arch or the animal is obese. Note any irregularity to its surface contour or loss of its sharp edges. Note the size of the spleen, if palpable.

Splenic masses are most frequently caused by neoplasia but also can be associated with immune-mediated diseases such as hemolytic anemia or thrombocytopenia. Gastric dilatation and volvulus may compromise venous drainage from the spleen and lead to splenic congestion.

Auscultation and Percussion

Not readily applicable to the examination of the lymphatic system.

DIFFERENCES IN CATS

The lymphatic system of the cat is very similar to that of the dog. Accessory lymph nodes are present in some cats. These include the accessory mandibular, accessory axillary, lateral retropharyngeal, and ventral superficial cervical. If present, they can be enlarged as a result of the same disorders that cause enlargement of the other peripheral lymph nodes.

RECOMMENDED READING

1. Evans HB, Christensen GC: Miller's Anatomy of the Dog, 2nd ed. Philadelphia, WB Saunders, 1979.

CLINICAL PROCEDURES

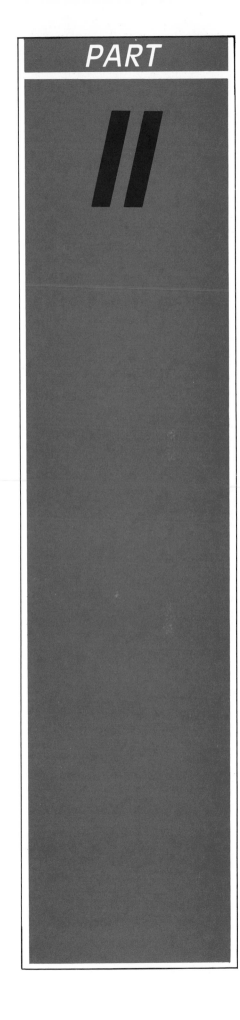

PART

II

Blood Collection

BARBARA H. McGUIRE

VENIPUNCTURE

Purpose of Procedure

1. To obtain a venous blood sample for diagnostic purposes
2. To gain access to a peripheral vein for intravenous injection

Complications of Venipuncture

1. Subcutaneous hematoma formation
2. Hemorrhage
3. Thrombosis of the vein
4. Phlebitis
5. Irritation of the skin at the site of needle penetration

Equipment Needed

1. Appropriately sized syringe and needle
2. Alcohol swab
3. Clippers and No. 40 clipper blade if necessary

Preparation

1. Selection of needle and syringe
   a. Jugular vein: A 20-gauge needle is most commonly used in large and medium-sized dogs whereas a 22-gauge needle is usually appropriate for small dogs and cats.
   b. Cephalic, saphenous, and femoral veins: A 20- or 22-gauge needle is usually adequate for larger dogs and a 22- or 25-gauge needle is used in smaller dogs and cats.
   c. Syringe selection: Syringe size is dictated by the volume of blood needed or material to be injected and the size of needle being used. Large volumes should not be injected into or withdrawn from the vein through small-gauge needles.
2. Selection of appropriate vein
   a. Venous blood samples: The jugular vein should be used whenever possible to obtain blood samples. Hemolysis or clotting of the sample is less likely owing to the larger size of needle that can be accommodated within the vein.
   b. Venous injection: Cephalic, saphenous, and femoral veins are most appropriate for injection techniques.
3. Skin preparation
   a. Clipping: If necessary, the hair over the venipuncture site can be clipped to allow better visualization of the vein. Owners should be informed prior to clipping.
   b. Alcohol swab: Wiping the venipuncture site with alcohol allows better visualization of the vein and removes gross contamination from the skin and hair.

Jugular Venipuncture

1. Positioning and restraint (Fig. 13–1)
   a. Place the animal in sternal recumbency on an examination table.
   b. With one hand, extend the neck vertically by grasping the muzzle and lifting the head.
   c. With the free hand, restrain the forelimbs by grasping the carpal joints and holding them firmly in front of the animal (Fig. 13–1B).

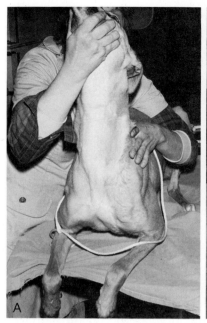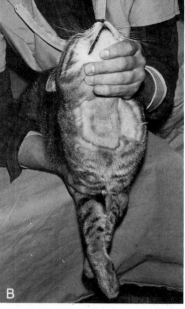

Figure 13–1. A, Position of dog for jugular venipuncture. B, Position of cat for jugular venipuncture.

d. *Note:* With large dogs, allowing them to sit upright on the floor is often easier than on a table. With some feline patients, over-restraint results in increased resistance to jugular venipuncture; try minimal restraint if struggling is excessive.

2. Venipuncture
   a. Distend the vein by placing pressure lateral to the trachea with the thumb of the free hand (Fig. 13–2).

   b. Trace the path of the vein from the angle of the mandible to the thoracic inlet, feeling for the distended vein.
   c. Insert the needle, bevel upward, at a 20- to 30-degree angle to the vein (Fig. 13–3). The needle should be inserted to the hub (except in small dogs and cats; see under Cephalic Venipuncture) to allow for stabilization within the vein.
   d. Withdraw the blood sample. Remove the

Figure 13–2. Jugular vein being distended with thumb of left hand while the index finger of the right hand identifies the vein.

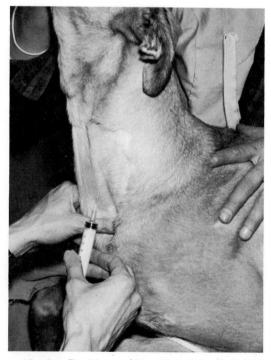

Figure 13–3. Position and insertion of needle into the jugular vein of a dog.

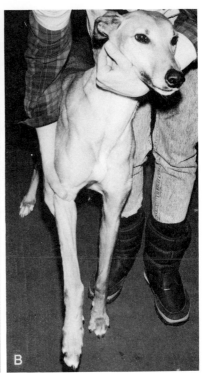

Figure 13-4. *A,* Position and restraint of cat for cephalic venipuncture. *B,* Position and restraint of large dog for cephalic venipuncture. The thumb is used to roll the vein into a dorsal position.

needle from the vein after pressure on the vein has been released.
  e. Place pressure over the venipuncture site immediately and hold for approximately 60 seconds.

Cephalic Venipuncture

1. Positioning and restraint (Fig. 13–4)
  a. Place the patient on the examination table in sternal recumbency (Fig. 13–4*A*).
  b. With one hand, restrain the head by grasping the muzzle and turning the head away from the leg to be used (Fig. 13–4*B*).
  c. With the other hand, grasp and stabilize the elbow from the lateral side and roll the vein dorsally to allow better visualization of the vein.
2. Venipuncture
  a. Stabilize the leg and skin over the vein with the free hand.
  b. Insert the needle as described previously, with at least 1 cm (0.5 cm in small dogs and cats) of the needle inserted into the vein.
  c. After withdrawal of the needle, a small gauze and tape wrap may be placed over the venipuncture site to prevent hemorrhage.

Saphenous Venipuncture

1. Positioning and restraint (Fig. 13–5)
  a. Place the animal in lateral recumbency

with the legs toward the venipuncturist and the back toward the assistant.
  b. Restrain the forelimbs and head by grasping the carpal joints and stretching the forelimbs forward while stabilizing the neck of the patient with the forearm of the same hand.
  c. Grasp the uppermost hind leg at the stifle joint to stabilize the leg and to distend the vein for venipuncture.
2. Venipuncture
  a. Grasp the hind leg at the tarsal joint to allow further stabilization.
  b. Insert the needle as described previously.
  c. After withdrawal of the needle, a small gauze and tape wrap may be placed over the venipuncture site.

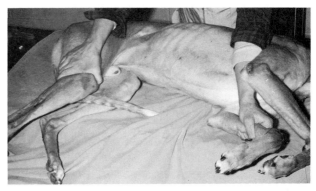

Figure 13-5. Position and restraint of dog for saphenous venipuncture. The right hand is used to restrain the hind limb and to distend and stabilize the vein.

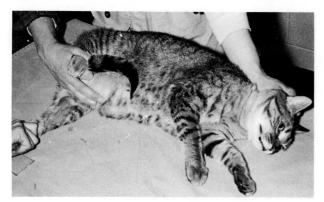

Figure 13–6. Position and restraint of cat for femoral venipuncture.

Femoral Venipuncture

1. Positioning and restraint (Fig. 13–6)
   a. This technique may require an additional assistant.
   b. Position the patient in lateral recumbency as described for saphenous venipuncture.
   c. Abduct and flex the uppermost hind leg, exposing the medial surface of the lowermost hind leg for venipuncture.
   d. Distend the vein by applying pressure to the proximal thigh.
2. Venipuncture
   a. With the free hand, grasp the leg at the tarsal joint.
   b. Insert the needle as described previously.
   c. After withdrawal of the needle, apply pressure to the venipuncture site for 60 seconds to prevent hemorrhage.

ARTERIAL PUNCTURE

Purpose of Procedure

1. To obtain an arterial blood sample for blood gas and acid/base evaluation

Complications of Arterial Puncture

1. Hemorrhage from puncture site
2. Thrombosis of the artery
3. Subcutaneous hematoma formation

Equipment Needed

1. 3-ml syringe
2. 25-gauge needle
3. Heparin
4. Gauze sponges, surgical scrub solution, and alcohol
5. Rubber cork from blood collection tube
6. Clippers and No. 40 clipper blade if necessary

Preparation

1. Preparation of syringe and needle
   a. Heparinize the 3-ml syringe by drawing heparin (1000 U/ml) into the syringe through the 25-gauge needle; then expel excess back into the bottle, leaving heparin only in the hub of the needle.
   b. Recap the needle and place the prepared syringe on a clean surface with the cork from the blood collection tube.
2. Selection of appropriate artery
   a. Available arteries include the femoral artery and the dorsal pedal artery.
   b. The femoral artery is most often used for arterial puncture. In patients that are difficult to restrain or grossly obese or when femoral puncture is not successful, the dorsal pedal artery is an alternative.
3. Skin preparation
   a. Clip excess hair from the puncture site.
   b. Surgically prepare the puncture site.

Femoral Arterial Puncture

1. Positioning and restraint (Fig. 13–7)
   a. Place the animal in lateral recumbency on an examination table.

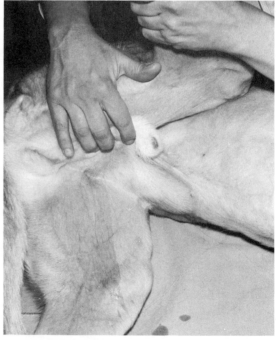

Figure 13–7. Position and restraint of dog for femoral arterial puncture.

b. Abduct and flex the uppermost hind leg to expose the inguinal region of the lowermost hind leg. Extend the lower hind leg.

c. In obese animals, it may be necessary to lift the caudal mammary glands or prepuce to expose the femoral artery of the lowermost leg.

d. *Note:* If the patient is in severe respiratory distress, placement in lateral recumbency may worsen its condition. Use of the dorsal pedal artery may be advisable in these patients.

2. Arterial puncture

a. Locate the femoral artery by palpating for a pulse.

b. Position the artery between the first and second fingers of the free hand (Fig. 13–8).

c. Insert the heparinized needle and syringe into the artery by piercing the skin lying between the fingers at a 60- to 90-degree angle (Fig. 13–9). Slowly advance the needle into the artery until blood appears in the hub.

d. Gently aspirate 1 to 1.5 ml of blood from the

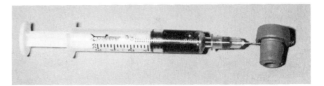

Figure 13–10. After expelling the air bubbles from the syringe, insert the tip of the needle into a rubber cork.

artery and withdraw the needle from the artery.

e. Immediately have assistant apply direct pressure to the puncture site using a clean gauge sponge. Pressure should be maintained continually for 5 minutes, and longer if necessary.

f. After withdrawing the needle from the artery, immediately expel air bubbles from the syringe and insert the tip of the needle into the rubber cork (Fig. 13–10). This plugs the needle and prevents exchange of gases between the blood and the atmosphere.

Dorsal Pedal Arterial Puncture

1. Positioning and restraint

a. Place the patient in sternal recumbency with the hind legs to one side.

b. Extend and stabilize the lowermost hind leg by grasping the distal tibia.

2. Arterial puncture

a. Palpate for the dorsal pedal artery along the dorsal surface of the hock and proximal metatarsal area. The artery is superficial and runs slightly medial to the midline of the leg (Fig. 13–11).

b. Proceed with arterial puncture as described above for the femoral artery. The angle of entry into this artery is 15 to 30 degrees and, therefore, the needle is more parallel to the skin.

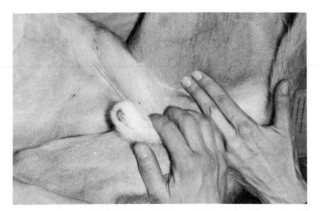

Figure 13–8. Locate the position of the artery by using the first and second fingers of the free hand.

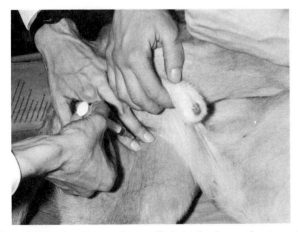

Figure 13–9. Insert the needle into the femoral artery at a 60- to 90-degree angle between the two fingers that are stabilizing the artery.

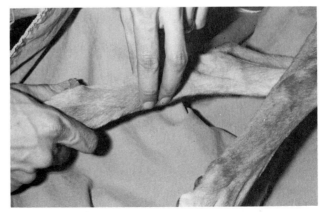

Figure 13–11. Position and restraint of dog for dorsal pedal arterial puncture.

Injection Techniques

Purpose of Procedure

1. To deliver a substance or medication parenterally

Complications of Injections

1. Hemorrhage at injection site
2. Hematoma formation
3. Irritation of local nerves, primarily with intramuscular injection
4. Irritation or necrosis of local tissue due to extravascular leakage of irritating substances with intravenous injection (e.g., thiopental, BSP, thiacetarsamide)

Equipment Needed

1. Needle and syringe of appropriate size (see below)
2. Alcohol swab
3. Clippers and No. 40 clipper blade if necessary
4. Tape and gauze bandage if injection is intravenous

Preparation

1. Selection of needle and syringe
    a. Needle selection: Needle size is determined by the size of the animal and the volume of material to be injected. In a large dog, a 20-gauge needle can be used for most peripheral veins and for intramuscular and subcutaneous injections. In smaller dogs and cats, a 22- or 25-gauge needle is more appropriate.
    b. Syringe selection: The size of the syringe is determined by the volume of material to be injected.
2. Preparation of medication
    a. Prior to giving any medication, make sure that the dosage, route, and time of treatment are correct. The patient should also be properly identified.
    b. Using sterile technique, place the needle onto the syringe.
    c. Wipe the top of the medication bottle with an alcohol swab.
    d. Invert the bottle and insert the needle into the rubber stopper.
    e. Slowly withdraw the desired amount of medication. If bubbles are present in the syringe or the hub of the needle, hold the syringe vertically with the needle dorsal and tap the syringe to force the bubbles to the top of the syringe. Eject the air through the needle (Fig. 14–1).

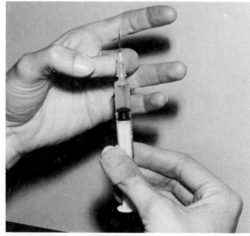

Figure 14–1. Removal of air bubbles prior to intravenous injection.

3. Patient preparation and restraint
   a. The patient should be restrained as necessary to allow for safe administration of medication. The assistant should hold the patient with the injection site exposed and head held away from the administrator.
   b. The injection site should be swabbed with alcohol as described in an earlier chapter.

INTRAVENOUS INJECTION

1. Selection of vein
   a. Dogs: The cephalic and saphenous veins are most often used in dogs for intravenous injection. The jugular vein should *not* be used, as extravascular injection is difficult to detect and the vein is hard to stabilize for injection.
   b. Cats: The cephalic and femoral veins are most appropriate for intravenous injection in the cat. As in the dog, the jugular vein should be avoided.
2. Injection
   a. Have the assistant distend the vein as described for venipuncture.
   b. With the needle at a 20- to 30-degree angle to the skin, insert the needle into the vein. Advance the needle into the vein to ensure stability (at least 1 cm in larger animals and 0.5 cm in small dogs and cats).
   c. Aspirate to test placement of the needle. A flash of blood should appear in the hub of the syringe.

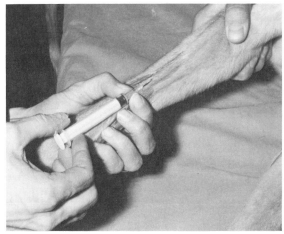

Figure 14-2. Stabilization of syringe for intravenous injection.

d. Have assistant release pressure on the vein.
e. Stabilize the syringe by holding the hub of the needle or barrel of the syringe between the thumb and forefinger, with the fingers wrapped around the limb (Fig. 14-2).
f. Inject the material at a moderate rate. Watch the injection site for swelling, which would indicate extravascular injection.
g. If a large volume of medication is to be injected, a periodic check of needle placement is appropriate. Redistend the vein and aspirate a small amount of blood to ensure continued placement in the vein.
h. Withdraw the needle from the vein. Apply direct pressure or place a gauze and tape bandage over the venipuncture site if needed.
i. Record the injection in the medical record.

INTRAMUSCULAR INJECTION

1. Selection of injection site
   a. Dogs: In large dogs, the semimembranosus and semitendinosus (hamstring) muscle groups are often used. The lumbar paraspinal muscles and quadriceps and triceps muscle groups are alternatives.
   b. Cats: In cats, the "hamstring" muscle group is smaller, and inadvertent nerve irritation or subcutaneous injection is more likely than in dogs. For this reason, the lumbar paraspinal and triceps muscles are often used.
   c. When giving multiple or frequent injections, rotate between the left and right sides and among different sites to prevent excessive soreness.
2. Injection
   a. Semimembranosus/semitendinosus injection: Grasp the muscle bodies between the thumb and forefinger of the free hand. Enter the muscle laterally, aiming in a slightly caudal direction to avoid the sciatic nerve (Fig. 14-3). Proceed with step d below.
   b. Lumbar paraspinal injection: Enter the paraspinal muscles in the midlumbar region, approximately 1 to 2 cm lateral to the

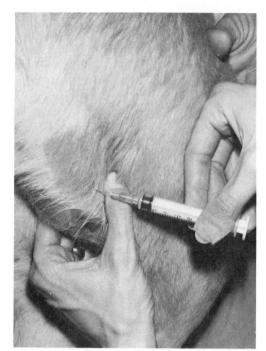

Figure 14-3. Hamstring injection.

dorsal spinous processes, depending on the size of the patient (Fig. 14-4). Proceed with step d below.

c. Quadriceps or triceps injection: Grasp the muscle bodies between the thumb and forefinger. Enter the muscle at an angle perpendicular to the femur (quadriceps) or humerus (triceps), aiming slightly caudally (quadriceps) or cranially (triceps).

d. Retract the plunger slightly to ensure against vessel penetration. A flash of blood appears in the hub of the needle if this has occurred. Replace the needle in a new site if a flash of blood is obtained.

e. Inject the medication at a moderate rate.

f. Withdraw the needle from the muscle.

g. Record the injection in the medical record.

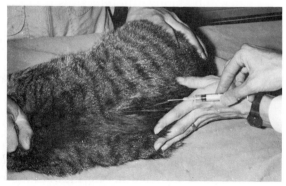

Figure 14-4. Paraspinal injection.

SUBCUTANEOUS INJECTION

1. Selection of injection site
   a. In both cats and dogs, the dorsal thoracic area is most commonly used for subcutaneous injection.
   b. If multiple injections are required, rotate between left and right sides and move slightly cranially and caudally to avoid excessive irritation.
2. Injection
   a. With the free hand, grasp the skin between the thumb and fingers, lifting the skin to form a fold.
   b. Insert the needle into the skin in the ventral part of the fold (Fig. 14-5).

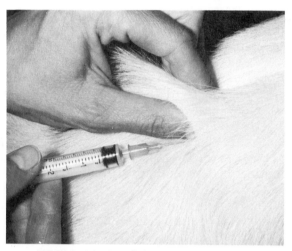

Figure 14-5. Subcutaneous injection.

c. Retract the plunger slightly to be sure a vessel has not been entered.

d. Inject the medication.

e. Withdraw the needle from the skin.

f. Record the injection in the medical record.

INTRADERMAL INJECTION

1. Selection of injection site
   a. This technique is used primarily for intradermal skin testing or for intradermal infiltration of anesthetic for minor procedures. The selection of injection site, therefore, depends on the purpose of the injection.
   b. The selected site should be clipped to allow for visualization of needle placement.

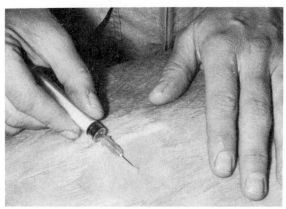

Figure 14–6. Intradermal injection.

2. Injection
   a. With the bevel of the needle facing upward, hold the syringe almost parallel to the skin, at a 5- to 10-degree angle.
   b. With the free hand, stretch the skin between the thumb and forefinger.
   c. Insert the needle into the skin just deep enough to cover the bevel (Fig. 14–6). The bevel can often be visualized through the skin with correct needle placement.
   d. Inject the material (usually 0.05 to 0.1 ml). A bleb of fluid can be seen or palpated within the skin with correct placement.
   e. Withdraw the needle from the skin.
   f. Record the injection in the medical record.

Intravenous Catheters

Purpose of Procedure

1. To gain continuous access to a peripheral vein for administration of fluids, blood products, anesthetic agents, or medication
2. To gain access to a peripheral vein for multiple blood samples
3. To gain access to the jugular vein for monitoring of central venous pressure

Complications of Intravenous Catheters

1. Phlebitis and thrombophlebitis
2. Thromboembolism
3. Hemorrhage
4. Subcutaneous placement and subsequent infiltration of material into the subcutaneous space
5. Air embolism

Equipment Needed

1. Clippers and No. 40 clipper blade
2. Surgical scrub and alcohol
3. Sterile gauze sponges
4. Bandaging material: sterile gauze sponges, gauze bandage, 1-inch adhesive tape, antimicrobial ointment
5. Injection cap
6. 3-ml syringe with heparinized saline
7. Appropriate catheter (see below)
8. Fluid administration set and extension tube if needed

Catheter Selection

1. General purposes
   a. *"Butterfly" winged infusion set:* This catheter is used for temporary or short-term access to a vein. It is not intended to stay in place beyond administration of intravenous medication but allows safe administration of larger volumes of medication or of medication that is irritating perivascularly without having to place a more longterm catheter. It is also useful for shortterm emergency fluid treatment in patients that are extremely shocky or dehydrated, as it can often be placed easily into a collapsed vein.
   b. *Over-the-needle catheter:* This is a useful catheter for short-term fluid therapy or treatment. This type of catheter should not be left in place for longer than 24 to 48 hours, as there is a greater risk of infection than with the through-the-needle catheter. It is, however, a catheter that is relatively inexpensive and easy to place.
   c. *Through-the-needle catheter:* This is the catheter of choice for long-term fluid therapy or intensive care treatment. With jugular placement, it can be used to monitor central venous pressure. It can be left in place for 3 to 4 days if correctly monitored and maintained.
2. Catheter size selection (Table 15–1)

Table 15–1
CATHETER SIZE SELECTION

Catheter Type	Animal	Vein	Size
"Butterfly" winged infusion set	Cat	Cephalic or femoral	22 or 23 gauge
	Dog	Cephalic or saphenous	20 or 22 gauge
Over-the-needle	Cat	Cephalic or femoral	20 or 22 gauge 1½ inch
	Dog	Cephalic or saphenous	18 or 20 gauge 1½ inch
Through-the-needle	Cat	Cephalic, femoral, or jugular	19 or 20 gauge 6 or 8 inch
	Dog	Cephalic or saphenous	19 or 20 gauge 8 or 12 inch
		Jugular	16 or 19 gauge 8 or 12 inch

Positioning and Restraint

The patient should be securely restrained as described for venipuncture, with the selected vein exposed.

Preparation

1. Wash hands well.
2. Widely clip the hair from the area of catheter placement.
3. Surgically scrub the vein and surrounding area, followed by swabbing with alcohol wipes.
4. Spray the prepared area with an antimicrobial solution.
5. In patients requiring catheter placement for more than 24 hours, the catheter should be placed with sterile gloves.

Catheter Placement

1. Butterfly (winged infusion) catheter
   a. Distend the vein by occlusion.
   b. Hold the catheter by folding the "wings" together between the thumb and index finger with the bevel of the needle upward (Fig. 15–1).
   c. Insert the needle into the skin over the vein at a 20- to 30-degree angle.
   d. Advance the needle into the vein up to the hub (or to a depth of 0.5 cm in small dogs and cats). A flash of blood appears in the tubing if the needle has entered the vein.
   e. Release the pressure on the vein.
   f. Flush the catheter with heparinized saline.
   g. Tape the catheter into place by placing 1-inch tape across the "wings" perpendicu-

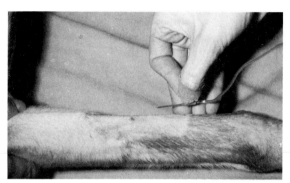

Figure 15–1. Insertion of butterfly catheter.

lar to the needle and around the patient's leg. Include a loop of the plastic tubing in the tape to prevent movement of the needle (Fig. 15–2).
   h. Proceed with administration of medication or fluid. Occasionally check the placement of the catheter by gentle aspiration of the syringe. A flash of blood should appear if placement is maintained.
   i. Record treatment time and location in the patient's record.

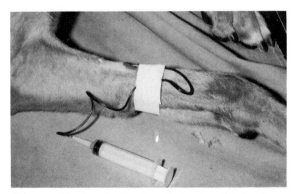

Figure 15–2. Butterfly catheter taped into place.

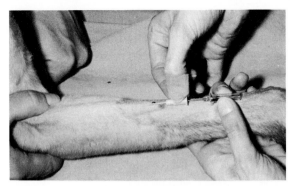

Figure 15–3. Advancement of over-the-needle catheter into vein.

2. Over-the-needle catheter
   a. Distend the vein by occlusion.
   b. With the bevel upward, advance the needle and catheter through the skin at a 20- to 30-degree angle and into the vein. The catheter and needle should be at least 0.5 cm into the vein at this point. A flash of blood appears in the hub of the needle if placement is correct.
   c. While holding the hub of the needle stationary with the thumb and forefinger of one hand (Fig. 15–3), thread the catheter into the vein — in larger animals, until the hub is at the point of skin penetration. This ensures that the catheter is adequately advanced to prevent subcutaneous leakage of medication.
   d. Withdraw the needle from the catheter and attach the injection cap to the catheter hub.
   e. Flush the catheter with heparinized saline.
   f. Tape the catheter to the limb by creating a tape "butterfly" around the catheter hub (Fig. 15–4) and encircle the limb.
   g. Apply a small amount of antibacterial ointment to a sterile gauze square and

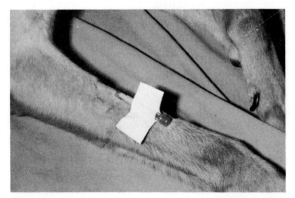

Figure 15–4. Tape "butterfly" around over-the-needle catheter.

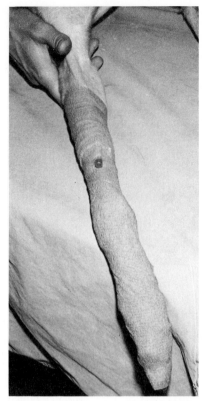

Figure 15–5. Completed placement of over-the-needle catheter.

place it over the site of skin penetration.
   h. Wrap the entire lower leg using stretch gauze and adhesive tape, leaving the injection cap exposed for easy access (Fig. 15–5).
   i. Flush the catheter with heparinized saline every 6 to 8 hours when not in use.
   j. Record placement time and location in the patient's record.

3. Through-the-needle catheter
   a. For jugular placement, the patient should be placed in lateral recumbency with the neck and head extended (Fig. 15–6). Have an assistant distend the vein by occlusion. Palpate for the vein in the jugular furrow, running between the thoracic inlet and the angle of the mandible. For cephalic or saphenous placement, restrain as previously described in Chapter 13.
   b. Remove the needle cover. Check to be sure that the catheter is fully withdrawn into the needle.
   c. Penetrate the skin with the bevel upward. For jugular placement, tent the skin as for a subcutaneous injection. This prevents accidental premature penetration of the vein.

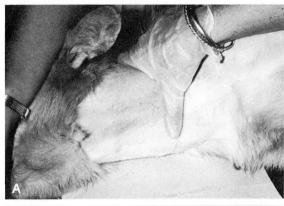

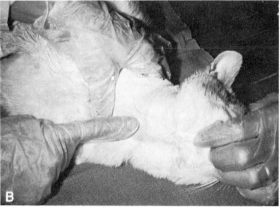

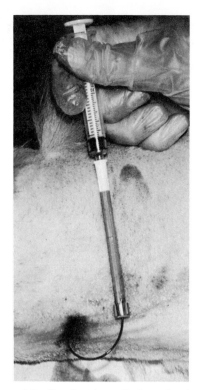

Figure 15-8. Jugular catheter prior to wrap.

Figure 15-6. Position for jugular catheter. *A,* Dog. *B,* Cat.

d. Enter the vein with the needle. A distinct "pop" is often felt and a flash of blood appears in the catheter tubing if penetration is successful. Advance the needle 0.5 cm into the vein.

e. Seat the end of the catheter securely into the needle hub (Fig. 15-7) and withdraw the needle from the skin.

f. Cover the needle with the needle guard and remove the plastic cover from the catheter tubing.

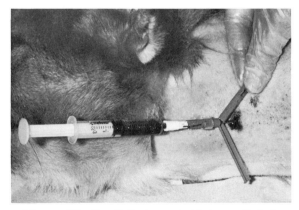

Figure 15-7. Catheter seated into needle hub.

g. Remove the wire stylet from the catheter (if present) and flush the catheter with heparinized saline.

h. Withdraw approximately 4 cm of the catheter from the vein and form it into a U-shaped loop. For jugular placement, the covered needle should lie perpendicular to the vein, pointing dorsally (Fig. 15-8). For limb placement, the covered needle should lie parallel to the limb.

i. Cover the loop and point of insertion with antibacterial ointment and sterile gauze sponges.

j. Tape the catheter into place using 1-inch adhesive tape encircling the covered needle first and then the neck or limb.

k. Using stretch gauze, gently wrap the limb or neck, leaving the injection cap of the catheter exposed.

l. Apply adhesive tape over the gauze to finish the wrap. When a limb is used, the entire leg and foot below the catheter should be wrapped (Fig. 15-9). For jugular placement, the wrap should be adequate to prevent significant movement of the catheter (Fig. 15-10).

m. Record placement time and location in the patient's record.

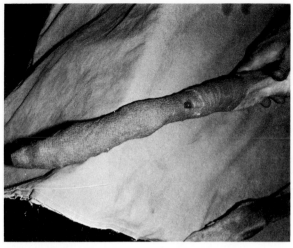

Figure 15 – 9. Completed placement and wrapping of cephalic catheter.

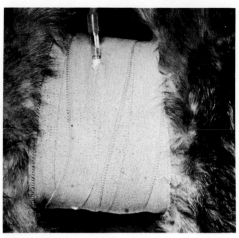

Figure 15 – 10. Completed placement and wrapping of jugular catheter.

Oral Administration

BARBARA H. McGUIRE

Purpose of Procedure

1. To administer medication or other substances via the oral cavity

Complications of Procedure

1. Accidental aspiration of medication into the respiratory tract
2. Decreased accuracy of dosage, particularly with liquid medication
3. Possible injury to patient or bite to administrator

Equipment Needed

1. Capsule/tablet: A small hemostat forceps is needed for the forceps technique.
2. Liquid: A dropper or syringe is needed for liquid medication.

Procedure

1. Capsule/tablet, finger method
   a. Grasp the tablet between the thumb and forefinger.
   b. With the free hand, gently grasp the maxilla of the patient and point the muzzle dorsally (Fig. 16–1).
   c. Open the mouth of the patient using the last three fingers of the hand holding the tablet. Keep the patient's nose pointed dorsally.
   d. Place the tablet at the base of the tongue and quickly close the mouth.
   e. Stroke the throat of the patient and/or blow on its nose to encourage swallowing of the tablet.
   f. Watch the patient closely for a few minutes

to ensure that the medication was swallowed.
   g. *Note:* In the cat, avoid placing the fingers of the free hand into the mouth, as this is very objectionable to most felines. Instead, drop the tablet into the back of the mouth without inserting the fingers (Fig. 16–2).
2. Capsule/tablet, forceps technique
   a. Grasp the tablet or capsule with a small hemostat.
   b. Follow steps b to f above.
3. Liquid medication
   a. Draw the medication into the provided dropper or appropriately sized syringe.
   b. Holding the muzzle with the free hand, point the nose slightly dorsally.

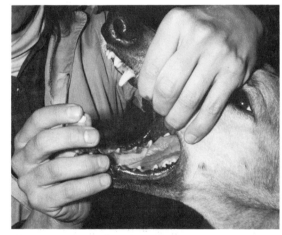

Figure 16–1. To open the mouth of a dog, grasp the maxilla posterior to the upper canine teeth and with the free hand use the last three fingers to keep the mandible open. The tablet is held between the index finger and thumb.

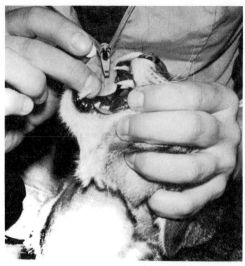

Figure 16–2. In the cat, the mouth is opened by inserting the fingers from over the maxilla posteriorly to the upper canine teeth. The tablet is dropped into the back of the mouth without inserting the fingers.

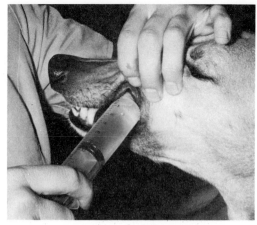

Figure 16–3. Placement of syringe into the lateral cheek pouch of a dog.

c. Place the end of the dropper or syringe into the lateral cheek pouch (Figs. 16–3 and 16–4).

d. Inject the medication into the pouch at a moderate rate, holding the mouth closed until the patient has started to swallow.

e. *Note:* In cats, liquid medication may need to be given in the back of the mouth (similar to the procedure for a tablet) rather than in the cheek pouch.

f. Record time and amount of medication given in the patient's medical record.

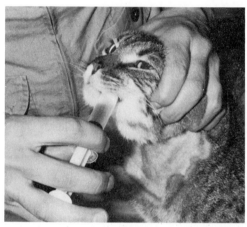

Figure 16–4. Placement of syringe into the lateral cheek pouch of a cat.

Impression Smears

BARBARA H. McGUIRE

Purpose of Procedure

1. To obtain a sample of cells from solid tissue for cytologic examination
2. To be able to differentiate between different types of solid tissue masses for therapeutic and diagnostic purposes

Equipment Needed

1. Scalpel blade
2. Paper towel
3. Thumb forceps
4. Glass slides

Procedure

1. Using a clean scalpel blade, cut into the tissue or biopsy mass to be examined, creating a fresh surface.

2. Pick up the tissue with the thumb forceps and blot the freshly cut surface on the paper towel, removing any fluid or exudate (Fig. 17–1). If a mass in situ is to be examined, blot it in a similar fashion with a sterile gauze sponge.

3. Gently touch the blotted surface to the face of a clean glass slide and remove quickly (Fig. 17–2). Three or four impressions can be made on a single slide.

4. Rapid drying of the impression smear can be accomplished by gently waving the slide in the air. This aids in preservation of both the cells and the quality of the slide.

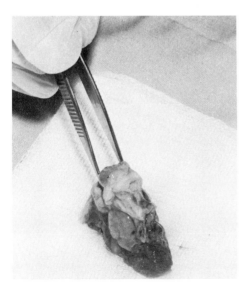

Figure 17–1. Blotting biopsy specimen.

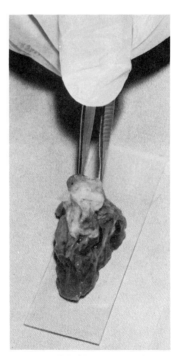

Figure 17–2. Making impression smear.

Fine-Needle Aspiration Biopsy

Purpose of Procedure

1. To obtain a sample of cells from an accessible mass for cytologic examination
2. To help differentiate among inflammation, neoplasia, and hyperplasia of organs such as lymph nodes or mammary glands
3. To help differentiate among inflammation, neoplasia, and hyperplasia of skin, subcutaneous, or other superficial masses

Complications of Procedure

1. Hemorrhage
2. Infection

Equipment Needed

1. 22-gauge needles, length determined by the depth of the mass to be sampled
2. 6-ml syringe
3. Glass slides
4. Surgical scrub and alcohol for skin preparation

Procedure

1. Preparation
   a. Have the patient restrained to allow exposure of mass to be biopsied.
   b. Generally, cleansing of the skin with scrub and an alcohol wipe is adequate. If a body cavity is to be entered (e.g., splenic aspiration), the hair should be clipped and a surgical scrub performed.

2. Aspiration biopsy
   a. Attach the needle firmly to the syringe.
   b. Grasp the mass between the thumb and fingers of the free hand.
   c. Insert the needle through the skin and into the mass.
   d. Apply negative pressure on the syringe (withdraw the plunger to the 3- to 5-ml mark) while the needle is still in the mass (Fig. 18–1). Gently release and reapply this negative pressure three or four times.

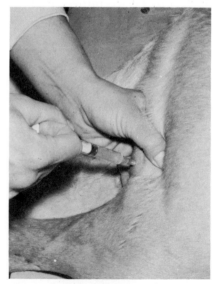

Figure 18–1. Position of needle and syringe for aspiration biopsy from the rear limb. Negative pressure is applied by withdrawing the syringe plunger while the needle is within the mass.

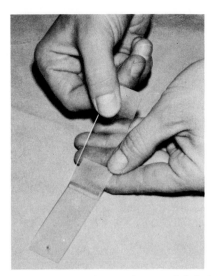

Figure 18-2. Aspirated liquid material being spread across the slide by a push slide technique.

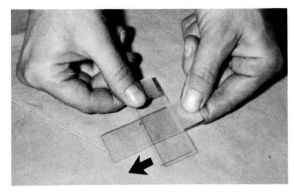

Figure 18-3. Aspirated viscous material being spread across the slide by a pull smear technique.

e. Release the negative pressure and quickly withdraw the needle from the mass.

f. Separate the needle from the syringe.

g. Retract the syringe plunger to the 3-ml mark; then reattach the needle.

h. Quickly eject the material in the needle onto a clean glass slide.

i. If the aspirated material is liquid, a push slide can be made (Fig. 18-2); if the material is more viscous, a pull smear should be made (Fig. 18-3).

Ear Care

EAR EXAMINATION

Purpose of Procedure

1. To complete a routine part of a thorough physical examination
2. To examine the external ear canal for possible inflammation, infection, foreign bodies, or masses

Complications of Procedure

1. Injury to the external ear canal
2. Injury to tympanic membrane

Equipment Needed

1. Otoscope
2. Appropriately sized otoscope cone

Procedure

1. Positioning and restraint
   a. Most patients will allow thorough examination of the external ear canal with good physical restraint. In very fractious animals or when the ear canal is severely inflamed or painful, care should be exercised in this examination. In some patients sedation may be required.
   b. Place the patient in sternal recumbency on an examination table.
   c. The assistant should be positioned opposite the examiner and should firmly grasp the muzzle of the patient from beneath with one hand and restrain the body of the patient from above with the other (Fig. 19–1).
2. Examination of the ear
   a. Examine the external pinna of the ear and note the presence of inflammation or exudate. Prior to use of the otoscope, determine which ear is more severely affected and examine the more normal ear first.
   b. Hold the otoscope in the same hand as the ear to be examined (e.g., left hand to examine the left ear) and grasp the external pinna of the ear with the free hand.
   c. Direct the cone downward into the vertical canal while applying gentle traction on the pinna (Fig. 19–2).

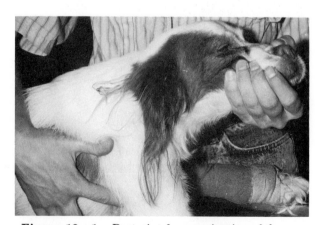

Figure 19–1. Restraint for examination of the ear.

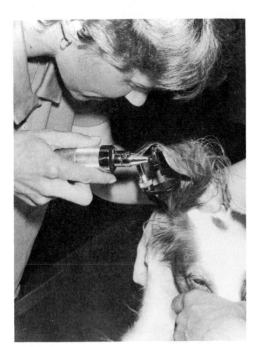

Figure 19–2. Examination of vertical canal.

d. When the opening of the horizontal canal is reached, slowly return the cone to a horizontal position so that the horizontal canal can be visualized (Fig. 19–3). At this point, the tympanic membrane should be visible at the end of the horizontal canal in most patients.

e. During the examination, note the presence of inflammation, exudate, or foreign bodies in the ear canal.

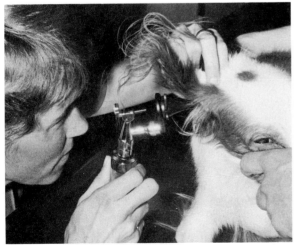

Figure 19–3. Visualization of horizontal canal and eardrum.

Purpose of the Procedure

1. To remove excess hair or cerumen from the external ear
2. To remove exudate present in otitis externa in order to facilitate treatment or to allow for more thorough examination of the external ear
3. To remove foreign bodies from the external ear

Complications

1. Increase (temporarily) in the inflammation present in the ear affected by otitis
2. Hemorrhage in the ear canal
3. Rupture of the tympanic membrane

Equipment Needed

1. Otoscope and appropriately sized cone
2. Ceruminolytic agent
3. Cotton
4. Bulb syringe
5. Antibacterial solution diluted 1:30
6. Cloth towel to catch cleaning solution from the ear
7. Cotton-tipped applicators
8. Glass slides and culturette (if cytology or culture is desired)
9. Hemostat forceps (if excess hair is present)

Procedure

1. Positioning and restraint
   a. See restraint for ear examination above.
   b. If the patient is fractious or if the inflammation of the external ear canal is severe or excessively painful, sedation, or even general anesthesia may be required. The safety of the patient and the thoroughness of the procedure should always be considered.
2. Cleaning
   a. If cytology or culture and sensitivity testing of the exudate is desired, this should be performed at this point, prior to cleaning.
   b. Excess hair in the canal, if present, can be removed by grasping the hair with a hemostat and gently twisting while applying traction (Fig. 19–4).

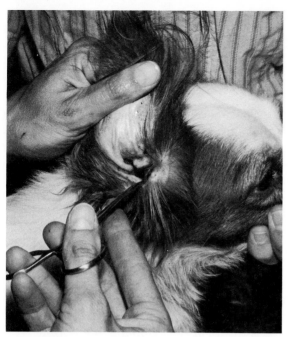

Figure 19-4. Removal of excess hair with hemostat.

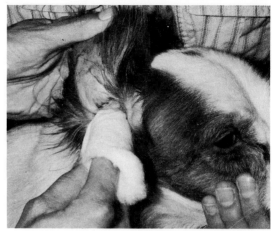

Figure 19-5. Wiping ear with cotton.

c. Place ceruminolytic agent into the ear and massage the ear at its base to distribute throughout the canal.

d. Fill the bulb syringe with dilute antibacterial solution, place the tip into the horizontal canal, and expel the liquid into the ear, using only moderate pressure. Massage the ear again.

e. Allow the fluid to drain out of the ear by tilting the head so that the ear is downward.

f. Gently wipe the ear with pieces of the roll cotton to remove the loosened exudate (Fig. 19-5). Cotton-tipped applicators should be used only sparingly and in the outer area of the ear. These can be irritating and potentially could cause rupture of the tympanic membrane if introduced too far into the canal.

g. Repeat steps c to f until no further exudate is present.

h. Using a clean otoscopic cone, examine the ear as described previously to assess the thoroughness of the cleaning and to look for previously unseen masses or foreign bodies. If a foreign body is present, carefully extract it using alligator forceps while visualizing the extraction through the otoscope.

i. Treat the ear with the appropriate medication by placing a few drops into the ear canal and massaging the ear.

Eye Care

BARBARA H. McGUIRE

TOPICAL MEDICATION

Purpose of Procedure

1. To apply medication to the surface of the bulb
2. To demonstrate the procedure to the client when dispensing ophthalmic medication (ointment or liquid)

Complications of Procedure

1. Irritation of conjuctiva
2. Trauma to the bulb

Ointment

1. Most patients can be medicated without the help of an assistant. If the patient is fractious or difficult, help may be needed for restraint.
2. The patient should be placed in sternal recumbency on an examination table.
3. Remove the cap from the appropriate tube of medication and express approximately ⅛ inch of medication from the tube. This forms a small "curly cue" on the tip of the tube.
4. With the index finger and thumb of the free hand, pull the patient's upper eyelid upward and the lower lid downward, away from the bulb. The third eyelid may prolapse slightly at this point.
5. Gently place the tip of the medication tube in the pouch formed by the lower lid. Deposit the medication in the space (Fig. 20–1).
6. Allow the lids to come together and gently massage the bulb through the lids to evenly distribute the medication.
7. Record the medication and the treatment time in the patient's medical record.

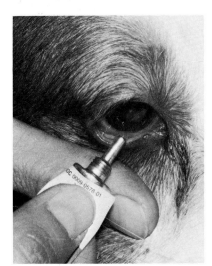

Figure 20–1. Placement of ointment in the lower lid pouch.

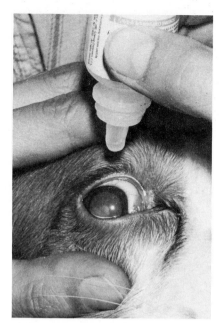

Figure 20-2. Placement of liquid medication in the eye.

Liquid Medication

1. Place the patient in sternal recumbency and lift the muzzle upward.
2. With the index finger and thumb of the free hand, separate the eyelids.
3. Holding the bottle of medication inverted 1 to 2 cm above the eye (Fig. 20-2), express two or three drops of liquid into the eye. It is not necessary to massage the eye, as liquid is easily distributed over the bulb.
4. Record the medication and treatment time in the patient's medical record.

SUBCONJUNCTIVAL INJECTION

Purpose of Procedure

1. To provide continuous medication of the eye via leakage through the needle puncture in the conjunctiva
2. To provide penetration of medication into the bulb

Complications of Procedure

1. Infection at injection site
2. Irritation at injection site
3. Inability to withdraw medication once given

Equipment Needed

1. Topical ophthalmic anesthetic drops
2. Tuberculin syringe with 25- to 27-gauge needle
3. Appropriate medication

Procedure

1. Place several drops of the topical ophthalmic anesthetic agent into the affected eye. Allow 3 to 5 minutes for the anesthetic to take effect. In fractious patients, sedation may also be necessary.
2. Have assistant restrain the patient's head.
3. Expose the bulbar conjunctiva by raising the upper eyelid.
4. With the bevel upward and the needle tangential to the bulb, insert the needle under the bulbar conjunctiva approximately 3 mm from the limbus (Fig. 20-3). The needle should be visible through the conjunctival membrane.
5. Inject the medication and withdraw the needle. A medication "bleb" should be visible under the conjunctiva.
6. Record the treatment and time in the patient's medical record.

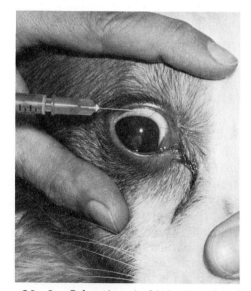

Figure 20-3. Subconjunctival injection of medication.

NASOLACRIMAL DUCT FLUSH

Purpose of Procedure

1. To test patency of nasolacrimal apparatus in cases of epiphora
2. To remove a foreign body or blockage if present

Complication of Procedure

1. Trauma or irritation to the eye or nasolacrimal puncta

Equipment Needed

1. Lacrimal cannula or blunted 22- to 25-gauge needle
2. Syringe, 6 or 12 ml, filled with normal saline
3. Topical ophthalmic anesthetic drops
4. Antibiotic-steroid ophthalmic drops

Procedure

1. Instill topical anesthetic into the affected eye or eyes. Allow 3 to 5 minutes for effect. In fractious patients, sedation may also be needed.

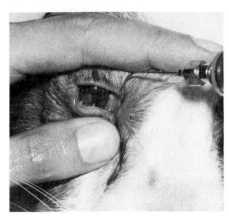

Figure 20–4. Flushing the nasolacrimal duct to remove an obstruction.

2. Introduce the cannula or blunted needle into the superior nasolacrimal puncta.
3. Inject saline into the duct. If fluid quickly appears in the ipsilateral nostril, the duct is clear.
4. If saline flows from the inferior puncta and not from the nostril, obstruction of the nasolacrimal duct is present. Apply digital pressure to the inferior puncta while injecting to attempt to dislodge the obstruction (Fig. 20–4). Often significant pressure is needed to clear the duct.
5. If flushing is successful, instill the antibiotic-corticosteroid drops into the eye or flush the medication through the cannula.

RECOMMENDED READING

Severin GA: Veterinary Ophthalmology. Colorado State University, College of Veterinary Medicine and Biomedical Sciences, 1982.

Urethral Catheterization

Purpose of Procedure

1. To obtain a urine sample for examination if cystocentesis is not successful or is contraindicated
2. To place a urinary catheter into the bladder for conditions in which an indwelling urinary catheter is indicated
3. To allow access to the lower urinary tract for radiographic studies (cystogram or urethrogram)

Complications of Procedure

1. Urethral or bladder trauma, irritation, or laceration
2. Urinary tract infection, especially with indwelling urinary catheters or in immunosuppressed patients

Equipment Needed

1. Sterile urinary catheter (Table 21–1)
2. Sterile lubricant (Surgilube, K-Y Jelly)

Table 21–1
GUIDELINES FOR SELECTION OF URETHRAL CATHETERS

Animal	Sex	Weight	Urethral Catheter*
Canine	Male	<20 lbs	3.5 French rubber or polyethylene urethral catheter
	Male	20–50 lbs	5 or 8 French rubber or polyethylene urethral catheter
	Male	>50 lbs	10 or 12 French rubber or polyethylene urethral catheter
	Female	<20 lbs	5 French metal, rubber, or polyethylene urethral catheter
		20–50 lbs	8 or 10 French metal, rubber, or polyethylene urethral catheter
		>50 lbs	10 or 12 French metal, rubber, or polyethylene urethral catheter
Feline	Male	All weights	3.5 French tomcat catheter
	Female	All weights	3.5 French tomcat catheter

* Selection of the appropriate catheter requires considerations other than patient weight. If a suggested catheter appears large for an individual animal or if urethral pathology is present, a smaller catheter may be needed.

3. Surgical scrub and saline or sterile water for rinse
4. 6- or 12-ml syringe for urine collection
5. Sterile gloves
6. Sterile saline for hydropulsion (obstructed male cat)
7. Indwelling catheters
   a. Urine collection bag or intravenous administration set with extension tubing
   b. 1-inch adhesive tape
   c. 3-0 nylon suture
   d. 22-gauge needle
   e. Antibacterial ointment

Preparation for Procedure

1. Most male and female dogs can be catheterized without sedation. Cats, both male and female, generally require tranquilization or general anesthesia for urethral catheterization. An exception to this would be the male cat that is toxic secondary to urethral obstruction. Caution should be exercised if tranquilization is used on these patients, as general depression and cardiovascular compromise are often present.

2. See individual catheterization techniques for further preparation.

Procedure

1. Urethral catheterization of the male dog
   a. Select a urinary catheter of appropriate size (Table 21–1).
   b. Measure the patient for proper placement of the catheter into the caudal bladder (Fig. 21–1). Note the distance on the catheter.
   c. Place the patient in lateral recumbency
   d. Extend the penis out of the prepuce.
   e. Gently wash the tip of the penis with sur-

gical scrub, followed by a saline or water rinse.
   f. Lubricate the tip of the urinary catheter with sterile lubricant.
   g. Wearing sterile gloves, advance the catheter into the urethra until correct placement is attained or urine is obtained. In some male dogs, slight resistance is felt at the level of the os penis or the prostate gland. Mild pressure is generally all that is required to overcome this resistance.
   h. If the placement is adequate but no urine is obtained, attach the syringe to the catheter and aspirate gently.
   i. Detach the syringe with the urine sample from the catheter prior to withdrawal of the catheter from the urethra.
   j. Withdraw the catheter from the urethra when the desired procedure is completed or suture into position for indwelling purposes (see procedure step 7 later in this chapter).
2. Urethral catheterization of the female dog—digital technique
   a. Select the urinary catheter of appropriate size (Table 21–1).
   b. Place the patient on an examination table with the hindquarters facing the clinician.
   c. The assistant should support the patient under the abdomen to prevent lowering of the hindquarters during catheterization (Fig. 21–2).
   d. Wash and rinse the vulvar and perineal areas.
   e. Lubricate the tip of the urinary catheter and the gloved finger of one hand.
   f. Insert the gloved and lubricated finger of

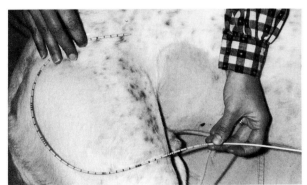

Figure 21–1. Measurement of catheter for placement in the male dog.

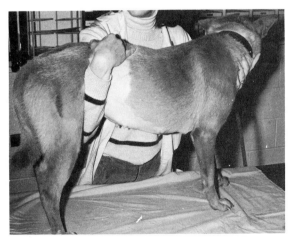

Figure 21–2. Restraint of the female dog for catheterization.

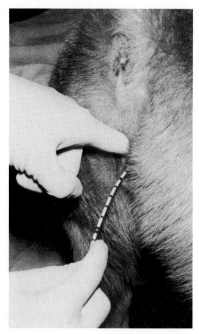

Figure 21-3. Insertion of catheter in digital technique.

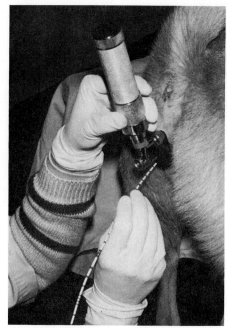

Figure 21-4. Visualization of the urethral papilla with the otoscope.

the free hand and palpate the urethral papilla on the vaginal floor. The papilla can be found 2 to 4 cm into the vagina in most dogs.

g. Leaving the finger placed on the urethral papilla, gently insert the urethral catheter under the finger and advance the tip to the urethral papilla (Fig. 21-3).

h. Thread the catheter into the urethra. The catheter should be palpable through the mucosa of the vaginal floor as it enters the distal urethra.

i. Advance the catheter until urine is obtained. If a metal urinary catheter is used, urine may be caught as it flows out of the end. A syringe may be attached to a rubber or plastic catheter to obtain urine.

j. Withdraw the catheter from the urethra or suture into position for indwelling purposes (see procedure step 7 later in this chapter).

3. Urethral catheterization of the female dog—otoscope technique

a. See procedure step 2 (digital technique), Steps a to d.

b. Place the sterile otoscope cone onto the otoscope.

c. Insert the otoscope cone into the vagina, using care to avoid the clitoral fossa. Insert the cone vertically, then straighten to horizontal when the pelvic canal is entered (Fig. 21-4).

d. Visualize the urethral papilla on the vaginal floor through the otoscope.

e. While still visualizing the papilla, thread the urethral catheter through the cone and into the urethra.

f. See procedure step 2, i and j.

4. Urethral catheterization of the male cat—unobstructed

a. Tranquilization or sedation is generally needed in the unobstructed male cat. Apply as necessary.

b. For short-term placement, the open-ended tomcat catheter is adequate. For indwelling purposes, a closed-ended tomcat catheter should be used. Select a catheter for placement and open the catheter cover, leaving the catheter in place (Fig. 21-5). Lubricate the end of the catheter with sterile lubricant.

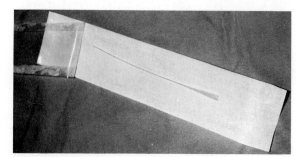

Figure 21-5. Opened tomcat catheter, sterility maintained.

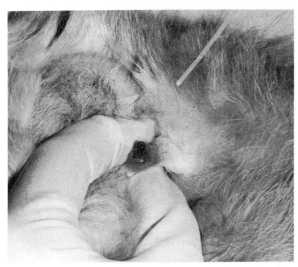

Figure 21 – 6. Exposed penis, prior to catheterization.

c. With the patient in lateral recumbency, retract the prepuce to expose the glans of the penis (Fig. 21–6). Gently wash the glans with surgical scrub and rinse.

d. After donning sterile gloves, insert the tip of the catheter into the urethral opening.

e. Gently thread the catheter into the urethra until urine is obtained or the catheter is fully threaded (Fig. 21–7).

f. If a urine sample is desired, attach a syringe to the end of the catheter or catch a sample as it flows from the end of the catheter. Withdraw the catheter from the urethra or suture into position for indwelling purposes (see procedure step 7 later in this chapter).

5. Urethral catheterization of the male cat—obstructed

a. As previously mentioned, care must be used when sedating the obstructed male cat. If depression exists, attempts should be made to catheterize the patient without sedation. If sedation is needed, the dosage of the medication should be adjusted to the minimum amount needed for the condition of the patient.

b. Select and open an open-ended tomcat catheter. Lubricate the tip of the catheter with sterile lubricant (see procedure step 4b).

c. Retract the prepuce and expose the glans of the penis. Gently wash and rinse the glans.

d. After donning sterile gloves, palpate the tip of the penis to check for the presence of a distal urethral plug or calculus. If an obstruction is present in the tip of the penis, gently massage the penis between the thumb and forefinger to attempt to dislodge the plug. If this is unsuccessful, proceed with the following steps. *Note:* When attempting retropulsion of a urethral calculus in an obstructed male cat, care must always be exercised, as use of excessive force or volume of fluid could result in significant urethral trauma or rupture of the urinary bladder.

e. Attach a 12-ml syringe filled with sterile saline to the open-ended tomcat catheter.

f. Insert the catheter into the urethral opening and thread the catheter into the urethra until the obstruction is reached.

g. Hold the syringe in one hand and compress the tip of the penis between the index finger and thumb of the other hand (Fig. 21–8). Gently inject a small amount of saline (1 to 2 ml) through the catheter, then release the pressure on the tip of the penis. If a flow of urine is obtained, proceed with

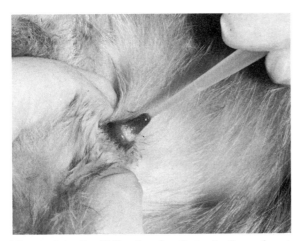

Figure 21 – 7. Fully placed catheter in the male cat.

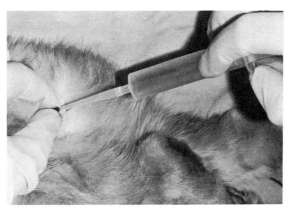

Figure 21 – 8. Retropulsion of urethral plug in the male cat.

threading the catheter into the bladder. If multiple obstructions are present, repeat the hydropulsion until the catheter is within the bladder and a flow of urine is obtained.

    h. Allow the bladder to empty. Obtain a urine sample if desired, then flush the bladder with sterile saline until the flush is clear. Do not overdistend the bladder.

    i. If an indwelling catheter is desired, the open-ended catheter should be removed from the urethra and a closed-ended catheter inserted. Suture into position as described in the final section of this chapter.

6. Urethral catheterization of the female cat

    a. Select appropriate urinary catheter (Table 21–1).

    b. Administer tranquilization or general anesthesia as indicated.

    c. Place patient in sternal recumbency.

    d. Wash perineal area with surgical scrub and rinse well.

    e. Wash hands and don sterile gloves.

    f. Have assistant restrain patient with the hind legs extended caudally over the edge of the examining table (Fig. 21–9).

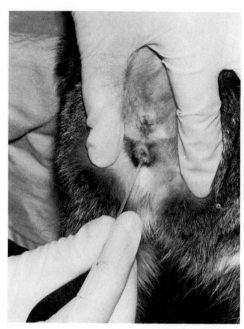

Figure 21–10. Insertion of catheter in female cat.

    g. Spread the vulvar lips with the free hand and insert the urethral catheter into the vagina (Fig. 21–10).

    h. Advance the catheter forward while staying on the midline. The urethral papilla is located approximately 0.7 to 1.0 cm within the vagina. The catheter should pass into the urethra with little resistance. If resistance is encountered, withdraw the catheter and start again. It is possible to force the catheter through the uterine stump and into the peritoneal cavity if the catheter does not enter the urethra and excessive pressure is used.

    i. If a urine sample is desired, attach a syringe to the catheter and aspirate or catch a sample as urine flows from the catheter.

    j. Withdraw the catheter when the procedure is completed, or suture into position for indwelling purposes (see procedure step 7 later in this chapter).

7. Placement and maintenance of indwelling urinary catheter

    a. Select the appropriate urinary catheter (Table 21–1). Polyethylene catheters are considered to be the best choice for indwelling purposes and should be used whenever possible. Examining gloves should be worn at all times for placement or handling of the collection system described below.

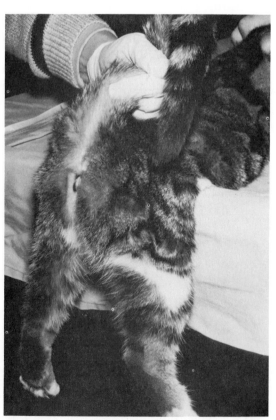

Figure 21–9. Restraint of the female cat for urethral catheterization.

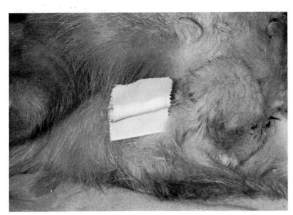

Figure 21–11. Tape "butterfly" for indwelling urethral catheter.

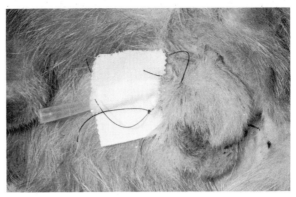

Figure 21–13. Catheter sutured in place.

b. Place catheter as described in previous sections.

c. Dry the exposed catheter.

d. Using 1-inch adhesive tape, place a "butterfly" on the catheter where it exits from the vulva or penis (Fig. 21–11).

e. Suture the butterfly to the prepuce or vulvar lips using 3-0 nylon suture. Suturing can be accomplished with little discomfort if a 22-gauge hypodermic needle is used rather than forceps and the suture needle. Pass the hypodermic needle through the skin of the prepuce or vulva. Thread the suture material through the needle, starting from the point (Fig. 21–12). Withdraw the needle from the skin and remove the needle from the suture. Tie the suture securely. Repeat on the other side of the butterfly (Fig. 21–13).

f. Aseptically attach a urine collection bag

with tubing or an intravenous administration tube to the end of the catheter.

g. Secure the catheter with tape to the tail or abdomen of the patient, leaving a sufficient amount of slack to permit movement without tension on the sutures and catheter.

h. If an intravenous administration set is used, place the distal end into a collection bottle. If venting is needed, insert a large-gauge needle into the rubber stopper to allow for urine flow (Fig. 21–14).

i. Place collection bottle below the patient,

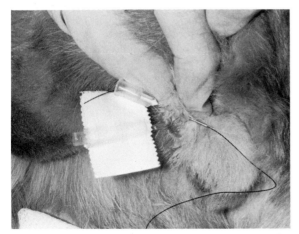

Figure 21–12. Threading of suture through hypodermic needle for indwelling catheter.

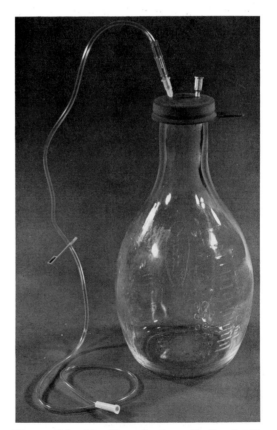

Figure 21–14. Vented urine collection bottle.

making sure there is enough tubing to allow for movement in the cage without tension on the system.

j. Place an Elizabethan collar on the patient if needed.

k. Place a strip of adhesive tape vertically on the bottle or bag and record the urine volume and time on the strip at regular intervals (three or four times a day).

l. Change the collection containers as needed and the entire collection system daily (excluding catheter).

m. Apply antibacterial ointment to the catheter exit site three times a day.

n. Keep the patient and environment immaculately clean at all times. All fecal material should be promptly removed from the cage.

Anal Sac Care

BARBARA H. McGUIRE

Purpose of Procedure

1. To empty anal sacs
2. To examine contents of anal sacs in cases of suspected anal sacculitis
3. To instill appropriate medication into infected anal sacs

Complication of Procedure

1. Possible rupture of impacted anal sac

Equipment Needed

1. Examination glove
2. Lubricant (petroleum jelly, surgical lubricant)
3. Roll cotton or gauze sponges
4. Cannulation syringe (curved tip)
5. Appropriate medication

Procedure — External Expression

1. Patient should be restrained in a standing position either on an examination table or on the floor. The assistant should support the patient under the abdomen to prevent the patient from sitting during the procedure.
2. Don the examination glove.
3. Gently raise the tail of the patient with the free hand to expose the anus.
4. Gently palpate the perirectal area to locate the anal sacs, located at approximately 4 and 8 o'clock to the anal opening (Fig. 22–1).
5. After locating the sacs, cover the anal opening with roll cotton or gauze.
6. Apply pressure dorsally and medially on each anal sac, using the index finger and thumb of the gloved hand (Fig. 22–2). Fluid expressed from the sacs should appear on the cotton or gauze as it is expressed from the anal sacs.
7. Examine the fluid for color and consistency and, if desired, make an impression smear of the fluid for microscopic examination.

Procedure — Internal Expression

1. Restrain patient as described in External Expression, Step 1.

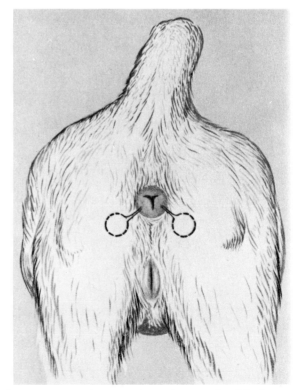

Figure 22–1. Anal sacs located at 4 and 8 o'clock to anus.

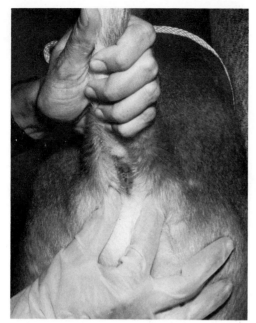

Figure 22–2. External expression of anal sacs.

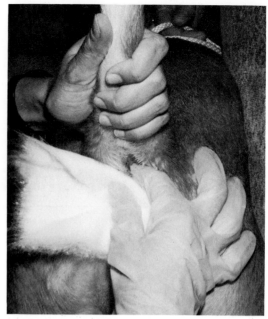

Figure 22–4. Internal expression of anal sacs.

2. Don examination glove and lubricate the index finger.

3. Insert the lubricated, gloved finger 2 to 3 cm into the rectum.

4. Locate one anal sac between the index finger within the rectum and the thumb externally (Fig. 22–3).

5. Cover the anal opening with cotton or gauze and express the anal sac between the thumb and index finger (Fig. 22–4). Repeat the procedure on the opposite anal sac.

6. Examine the fluid for color and consistency and, if desired, make an impression smear of the fluid for microscopic examination.

Procedure — Anal Sac Cannulation

1. Fill the cannulation syringe with 3 to 5 ml of medication.

2. Restrain the patient as described in External Expression, Step 1.

3. Lubricate the tip of the cannulation syringe.

4. Locate the opening of the anal sac at the mucocutaneous junction of the anus and insert the tip of the syringe 0.5 to 0.8 cm into the sac (Fig. 22–5).

5. Inject 1 to 2 ml of medication into the sac.

6. Repeat the procedure on the opposite side.

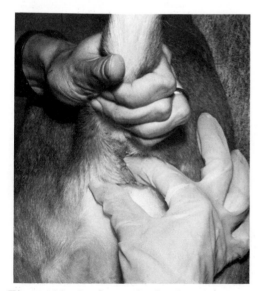

Figure 22–3. Internal palpation of anal sacs.

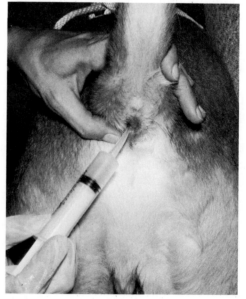

Figure 22–5. Cannulation of anal sac.

Enema Administration

BARBARA H. McGUIRE

Purpose of Procedure

1. To relieve constipation or obstipation
2. To evacuate the distal colon and rectum in preparation for radiographic studies (e.g., barium enema, urologic contrast studies)
3. To administer medication in specific medical conditions (e.g., betadine enema for hepatic encephalopathy)

Complications of Procedure

1. Rectal trauma, from mild irritation to rupture of the colon
2. Vomition, primarily in the cat, when too large a volume of fluid is administered rectally

Equipment Needed

1. Examination gloves
2. Lubricant
3. Enema administration bag (canine) or bulb syringe and bowl (feline)
4. Warm soapy water (Ivory or camomile), 5 to 10 ml/kg of body weight. In cases of obstipation, the addition of a water-soluble lubricant (K-Y Jelly or glycerine) may be helpful.

Note: In any *severely* obstipated patient, general anesthesia should be considered for purposes of removing the fecal material. This allows for improved relaxation of the rectal musculature and easier manipulation of fecal material.

Procedure

1. Canine
   a. Place the warm enema solution into the administration bag.
   b. The patient should be restrained in a standing position. If possible, administer the enema in an area appropriate for defecation, as enema results are often rapid. Large dogs should be placed in a run, whereas small dogs may be restrained on a drain table.
   c. Hang the enema bag in a convenient position above the patient (Fig. 23–1).
   d. Don the examination gloves.
   e. Lubricate the tip of the tubing.
   f. Insert the tip of the enema tubing into the

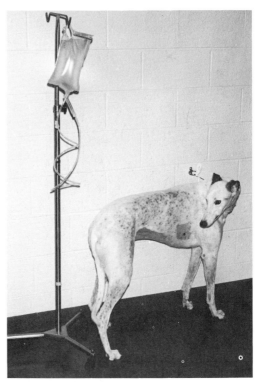

Figure 23–1. Hanging bag prior to enema.

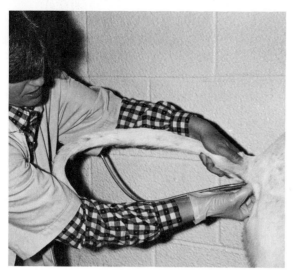

Figure 23–2. Compression of anal opening around enema tube.

patient's rectum; approximately 5 to 6 cm in large dogs and 2 to 3 cm in small dogs. Gently grasp the anus, placing pressure on the tubing (Fig. 23–2). This will prevent the enema fluid from immediately flowing out of the rectum.

g. Open the clasp on the enema tubing and administer the fluid.
h. Record the treatment and any results in the patient's record.

2. Feline
a. Place the measured fluid into the bowl.
b. The patient should be restrained on a drain table, either standing or in lateral recumbency.
c. Don the examination gloves.
d. Fill the bulb syringe from the bowl and lubricate the tip of the syringe.
e. Insert the tip of the bulb syringe into the rectum, approximately 1.5 to 2 cm.
f. Slowly compress the syringe while gently grasping the anus with the free hand. This will prevent the enema fluid from immediately flowing out of the rectum.
g. Repeat Steps d to f until the desired amount of fluid has been given. It is important to give the total volume relatively slowly (3 to 5 minutes), as rapid administration can result in vomition.
h. Record the treatment and any results in the patient's record.

Intubation

BARBARA H. McGUIRE

ENDOTRACHEAL INTUBATION

Purpose of Procedure

1. To gain access to the respiratory tract for ventilatory assistance and oxygen administration in the unconscious animal
2. To administer gas anesthetic agents
3. To allow for transtracheal aspiration in the cat (see Chapter 26)
4. For intratracheal administration of emergency drugs

Complications of Procedure

1. Oral, pharyngeal, or tracheal trauma due to the use of excessive force or improper technique or equipment
2. Hemorrhage or leakage of air into the surrounding tissue due to the above
3. Laryngeal spasm

Equipment Needed

1. Appropriate endotracheal tube (Table 24–1)
2. Sterile water-soluble lubricant
3. Laryngoscope, if available
4. 18 to 24 inches of gauze
5. A clean, empty 12-cc syringe
6. Gauze sponge
7. Mouth gag, if needed
8. Applicator stick (for intubation with an endotracheal tube of 4 mm or less)

Preparation for Procedure

1. Check the cuff of the endotracheal tube for leaks by inflating it fully with air. Deflate the cuff after inspection.
2. Sparingly lubricate the end of the tube and place it on a clean paper towel.

Procedure — Laryngoscopic Technique

1. Place the patient in sternal recumbency on the table.
2. Assistant should hold the patient's head up and open the mouth. Do not hold the head by the throat area, as distortion of the pharyngeal and laryngeal areas will result.

Table 24–1 GUIDELINES FOR SELECTION OF ENDOTRACHEAL TUBES IN THE CAT AND DOG		
Species	**Body Weight (kg)**	**Tube Size (Internal Diameter)**
Feline	1 to 2	3.0 to 4.0
	2 to 4	4.0 to 4.5
	>4	5.0
Canine	<5	5.0 to 7.0
	5 to 10	8.0 to 10.0
	10 to 20	11.0 to 12.0
	>25	12.0

Note: Always consider the individual patient when selecting an endotracheal tube. Variability of tracheal size exists; therefore, select the largest tube that can be introduced without force.

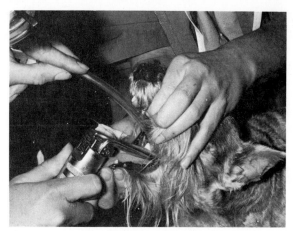

Figure 24–1. Laryngoscopic placement of endotracheal tube.

3. Grasp the tongue of the patient with one hand, using the gauze sponge if excess saliva is present.

4. Pull the tongue forward, extending the head and neck.

5. Introduce the laryngoscope into the mouth and guide the tip of the blade over the epiglottis (Fig. 24–1). The handle of the laryngoscope should be directed ventrally.

6. Ease the tip of the endotracheal tube between the arytenoid cartilages and into the larynx. If the tube does not pass with gentle pressure, try a smaller tube.

7. Advance the tube into the trachea until the cuff is just beyond the larynx (Fig. 24–2). If the tube is advanced too far into the trachea, inadvertent placement of the tube into a single mainstem bronchus could occur.

8. Attach the adapter of the endotracheal tube to the anesthetic machine or oxygen line as desired.

9. Inflate the cuff of the tube by attaching an empty syringe to the cuff port and injecting air into the cuff while squeezing the rebreathing bag on the anesthetic machine (pop-off valve closed). Inject only until no further air escape is heard. Open the pop-off valve. If no anesthetic machine is being used, fill the cuff until the "bubble" at the cuff port offers gentle resistance when squeezed between the thumb and forefinger. Do not overinflate the cuff, as this may cause trauma to and ulceration of the trachea.

10. Tie the length of gauze around the tube in a half hitch, just caudal to the adapter. Tie the gauze around the upper or lower jaw (dog) or behind the ears (cat).

Procedure — Visual Technique (No Laryngoscope)

1. Follow Steps 1 to 4 of the Laryngoscopic Technique.

2. Visualize the epiglottis, which should be pulled forward with the tongue. The laryngeal aperture will be visible (Fig. 24–3).

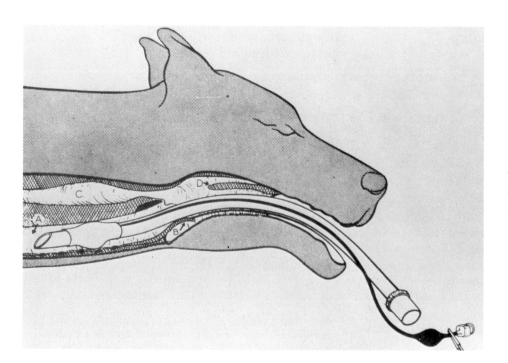

Figure 24–2. Correct placement of endotracheal tube. *A,* Trachea. *B,* Epiglottis. *C,* Esophagus. *D,* Soft palate.

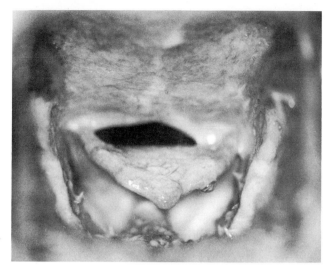

Figure 24-3. Visualization of larynx.

3. Pass the endotracheal tube between the arytenoid cartilages and into the trachea.

4. Complete Steps 7 to 10 of the Laryngoscopic Technique.

Procedure — Digital Technique (Dog Only)

1. Place the patient in right lateral recumbency.

2. Have the assistant hold the mouth open, or use a mouth gag if alone.

3. Using the right hand, grasp the tongue and pull it forward, extending the head and neck.

4. With the left hand, introduce the tube over the base of the tongue to where the tip of the tube is resting on the epiglottis.

5. Place the index finger of the left hand on top of the arytenoid cartilages and guide the tube into the larynx, pushing the tube forward with the right hand (Fig. 24-4).

6. Complete Steps 7 to 10 of the Laryngoscopic Technique.

Notes and Comments

1. Always deflate the cuff of an endotracheal tube prior to removal from the trachea.

2. Applicator sticks are sometimes inserted into the lumen of small endotracheal tubes to lessen their flexibility when intubating cats and small dogs. When the tube is passed into the trachea, immediately remove the applicator stick.

3. If there is any doubt of proper placement, double check to be sure that the tube is in the trachea. When bag ventilation is used, or air is blown into the tube, the chest should expand. When the chest is depressed, air can be felt being expelled from the tube. If the tube is not in the trachea, deflate the cuff and remove the tube. Try again!

CHEST TUBE PLACEMENT

Purpose of Procedure

1. To provide an avenue for repeated or continuous aspiration of fluid or air from the thoracic cavity

2. To allow access to the thoracic cavity for repeated lavage or intrathoracic administration of medication

Figure 24-4. Introduction of endotracheal tube, digital technique.

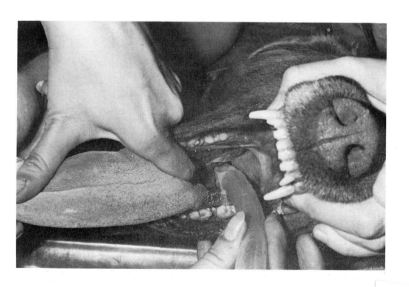

Complications of Procedure

1. Hemorrhage of skin or subcutaneous tissues at placement site
2. Laceration of lung tissue, resulting in hemorrhage and/or rupture of lung parenchyma
3. Destabilization of a patient in respiratory distress due to positioning in lateral recumbency for tube placement
4. Infection due to lack of asepsis during placement or maintenance

Equipment Needed

1. Sterile chest tube, preferably a commercial chest tube, 14 to 16 French. If a rubber tube or urethral catheter is used, cut three or four side holes near the end to provide better drainage. Sterility should be maintained.
2. Clipper and number 40 blade
3. Surgical scrub and alcohol, cotton balls
4. Cap, mask, and sterile surgical gloves
5. Minor sterile surgical pack:
   scalpel and blade
   scissors
   needle holders
   straight hemostat
   two curved hemostats or Carmalt forceps
   gauze sponges
6. Nylon suture material with needle, 2-0
7. Christmas-tree adapter
8. Three-way stopcock
9. 35- or 60-cc syringe
10. Intravenous extension tubing
11. Bandaging material:
    sterile gauze sponges
    antimicrobial ointment
    stretch gauze wrap
    stretch adhesive wrap
12. 2 percent lidocaine, 3-cc syringe, and 25-gauge needle

Preparation for Procedure

1. Except in very critical patients, sedation/analgesia is beneficial in order to maintain strict asepsis and to decrease the discomfort of the patient during chest tube placement. Medication such as meperidine, butorphanol, and oxymorphone is useful for this purpose. General anesthesia is often contraindicated in cases that require chest tube placement and should be used only if the patient is very stable and sedation is inadequate.
2. Place the patient in lateral recumbency.
3. Clip the lateral thorax from the fifth to the twelfth intercostal space.
4. Surgically prepare the clipped skin.
5. Infiltrate the skin and subcutaneous tissue over the mid–tenth intercostal space with lidocaine. Infiltrate an area of the intercostal muscles of the eight intercostal space, directly cranial to the previously infiltrated skin. The chest tube will enter the pleural cavity two intercostal spaces cranial to the skin incision (Fig. 24–5).
6. Don surgical cap, mask, and gloves and drape the prepared area with the sterile drape.

Procedure

1. Make a 1- to 2-cm incision in the skin over the infiltrated area of the tenth intercostal space.
2. Using the nylon suture material, preplace a purse-string suture around the incision (Fig. 24-6).

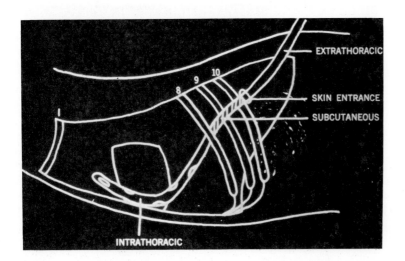

Figure 24–5. Skin incision and chest penetration location for chest tube placement.

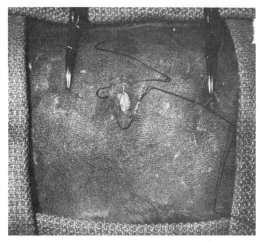

Figure 24–6. Preplacement of purse-string suture for chest tube placement.

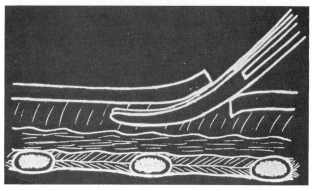

Figure 24–8. Creation of subcutaneous tunnel using curved hemostat.

Leave the ends of the suture loose and do not remove the needle from the suture.

3. Measure the tube to allow for adequate placement within the chest cavity and clamp the straight hemostat on the tube at the point of maximum insertion (Fig. 24–7), thus sealing the tube prior to placement.

4. Tunnel cranially through the subcutaneous tissue using the curved hemostat, curve facing the skin. The tunnel created should extend to the infiltrated area of the eighth intercostal space (Fig. 24–8).

5. Rotate the tip of the curved hemostat downward, and slowly force the tip through the intercostal muscles of the eighth intercostal space and into the pleural space (Fig. 24–9). Penetration should occur just cranial to the ninth rib in order to avoid the intercostal vessels and nerve located on the caudal surface of the eighth rib.

6. Spread the jaws of the hemostat slightly to enlarge the pleural opening a small amount.

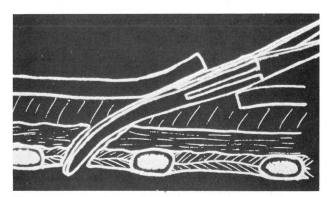

Figure 24–9. Penetration into pleural space with hemostat.

7. Grasp the tip of the chest tube with the second curved hemostat so that the tip of the tube is even with the tip of the hemostat.

8. Withdraw the hemostat that is in place in the chest; simultaneously insert the hemostat holding the chest tube into the subcutaneous tunnel (Fig. 24–10).

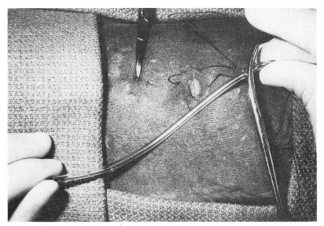

Figure 24–7. Measurement of tube for placement.

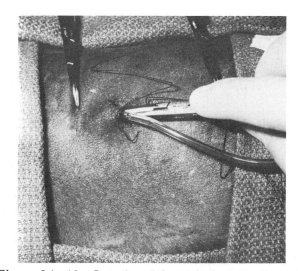

Figure 24–10. Insertion of chest tube/hemostat into subcutaneous tunnel.

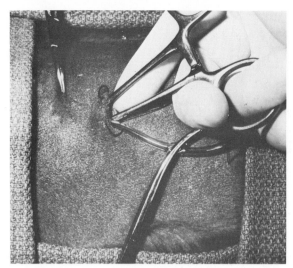

Figure 24–11. Advancement of chest tube/hemostat into pleural cavity.

9. Advance the hemostat tip and chest tube through the pleural opening and into the chest approximately 1 cm (Fig. 24–11).

10. Release the tube from the hemostat, withdraw the hemostat, and manually advance the tube into the chest up to the cross-clamp (see Step 3). **Do not remove the cross-clamp until instructed to do so.**

11. Tighten the purse-string suture around the tube and knot it securely. Do not cut off the ends of the suture.

12. Using 1-inch adhesive tape, place a tape butterfly around the tube between the cross-clamp hemostat and the skin entrance, then pass the needle and suture through the butterfly and knot again (Fig. 24–12). Cut off the excess suture material.

13. Using the remaining suture, secure the tape butterfly to the skin by placing a suture through each of the "wings."

14. Firmly attach the Christmas-tree adapter to the chest tube and then the extension tubing to the adapter. Place the three-way stopcock on the syringe and attach these to the extension tubing so that the final order is as follows: syringe, three-way stopcock, extension tubing, adapter, chest tube.

15. Close the three-way stopcock to the patient and close the clamp on the extension tubing.

16. The cross-clamp can now safely be removed from the chest tube.

17. Apply antimicrobial ointment to the skin at the tube entrance and cover with sterile gauze sponges. Wrap the chest with the stretch gauze followed by the elastic adhesive wrap. Include a loop of the extension tubing in one layer to prevent traction on the tube and include the syringe in the final layer of wrap (Fig. 24–13).

18. To aspirate from the chest tube, remove the outer layer of adhesive wrap, close the stopcock to the outlet, release the clamp on the extension tubing, and apply negative pressure on the syringe. To empty the syringe, close the stopcock to the patient and eject contents through the outlet. Repeat until no more aspirate is removed.

19. Close the stopcock to the patient, clamp the extension tubing closed, and replace the syringe under the wrap. Record the results of aspiration in the patient's record.

20. Apply Elizabethan collar to protect tubing and bandages.

Note: A patient with a chest tube in place should not be left unattended, owing to the possible development of pneumothorax. If a patient must be left alone, a hemostat clamp should be placed on the chest tube just beyond the butterfly and the clamp taped into the bandage. This clamp, in addition to

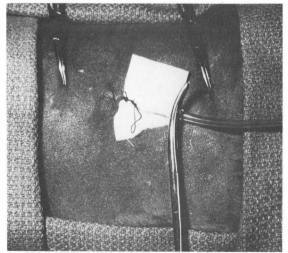

Figure 24–12. Tightened purse-string suture and secured butterfly on chest tube.

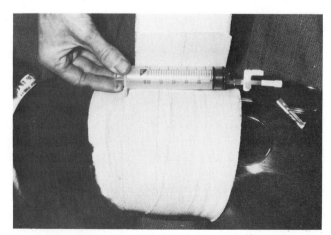

Figure 24–13. Final wrapping of chest tube.

the stopcock and extension tube clamp, provides a greater degree of safety to the patient.

NASOGASTRIC INTUBATION

Feline

Purpose of Procedure

1. To provide access to the gastrointestinal tract for purposes of nutritional support in patients suffering from anorexia or inability to ingest food

Complications of Procedure

1. Mild nasal hemorrhage due to trauma to the nasal turbinates
2. Mild nasal irritation due to the presence of the feeding tube
3. Incorrect location of the tube resulting in tracheal placement and subsequent aspiration of administered material

Equipment Needed

1. Infant feeding tube or red rubber tube; 5 French and 24 to 36 inches long
2. Nylon or silk suture with a cutting needle, 3-0
3. 1 to 2 cc of 2 percent lidocaine in a 3-cc syringe or ophthalmic anesthetic drops
4. Sterile water-soluble lubricant
5. 1-inch adhesive tape
6. 5 cc saline in a syringe
7. Elizabethan collar

Procedure

1. Place the patient on an examination table in sternal recumbency. If the patient is fractious, mild sedation may be needed for intubation. It is important, however, that the patient remain alert, as a strong swallow reflex is helpful to facilitate passage of the tube into the esophagus.
2. Point the nose of the patient dorsally and instill 1 cc of 2 percent lidocaine or several drops of the ophthalmic anesthetic into the nostril (Fig. 24–14).
3. Extend the neck of the patient and premeasure the length of tube to be passed (Fig. 24–15). The tip of the tube should extend to the mid-distal esophagus, as gastric placement results in increased incidence of vomition. Therefore, measure the dis-

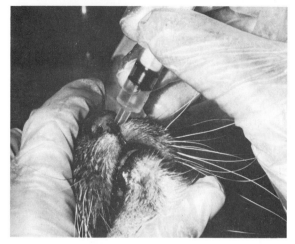

Figure 24–14. Instillation of local anesthetic into nostril for nasogastric intubation.

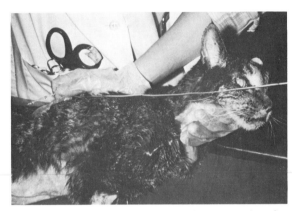

Figure 24–15. Premeasurement of nasogastric tube for placement.

tance to the midthorax and note the point on the tube.

4. Generously lubricate the tip of the tube with the water-soluble lubricant.
5. With the head firmly restrained, introduce the tip of the tube into the nostril, guiding the tube in a ventromedial direction (Fig. 24–16). This

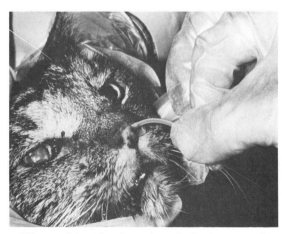

Figure 24–16. Insertion of tube into nostril.

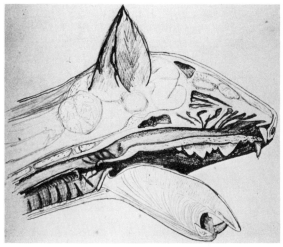

Figure 24–17. Diagram of ventral meatus and esophagus, feline.

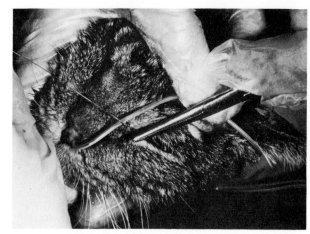

Figure 24–19. Placement of nasal suture for nasogastric tube.

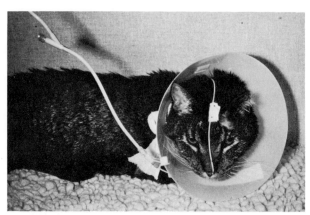

Figure 24–20. Nasogastric tube in place with Elizabethan collar.

allows placement into the ventral meatus, which is large in the cat and extends directly to the nasopharynx and esophagus (Fig. 24–17). If resistance is felt 1 to 2 cm into the nose, withdraw the tube and try again, as insertion of the tube into the dorsal meatus may have occurred.

6. Advance the tube into the esophagus to the predetermined point. As the tube is passed, the patient may swallow several times or gag mildly.

7. Attach the syringe containing the saline to the end of the feeding tube and inject the saline slowly (Fig. 24–18). If no coughing results, tracheal placement is unlikely.

8. Place a single suture in the skin of the nose and around the tube to anchor it in place. It is important that this suture be very close to where the tube exits from the nostril in order to prevent easy removal by the patient (Fig. 24–19).

9. Make a "butterfly" around the tube with 1-inch adhesive tape approximately 3 cm from the nostril. Suture the "butterfly" to the skin of the head between the ears.

10. Place the Elizabethan collar on the patient and exit the tube out the back of the collar (Fig. 24–20).

11. To ensure proper location of the tube, a lateral radiograph of the thorax should be taken. The tube should be visualized within the mid to distal esophagus.

Canine

Purpose of Procedure

1. To maintain decompression of the stomach of a dog with gastric dilatation
See *Feline Nasogastric Intubation.*

Complications of Procedure

See *Feline Nasogastric Intubation.*

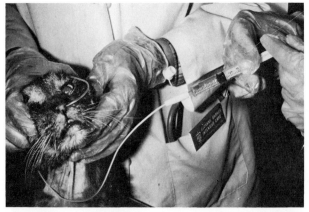

Figure 24–18. Injection of saline to check for tracheal placement.

Equipment Needed

1. Infant feeding tube or red rubber tube; 6 French and 36 inches long
2. See *Feline Nasogastric Intubation,* Equipment Needed, numbers 2 to 7.

Procedure

1. See *Feline Nasogastric Intubation,* Procedure, Steps 1 to 4.

2. Insert the tube into the nostril, initially heading slightly dorsally. This is necessary in order to advance the tube past the small ventral ridge found just inside the nostril in dogs. When the tip has passed the ridge, approximately 1 cm into the nostril, redirect the tube in a medioventral direction and advance the tube into the ventral meatus.

3. See *Feline Nasogastric Intubation,* Steps 6 to 11. In Step 9, the tape "butterfly" should be placed 3 to 7 cm from the nostril, depending on the size of the dog.

Dental Prophylaxis

Purpose of Procedure

1. Removal of subgingival plaque and calculus
2. Prevention of irreversible periodontal disease
3. Inspection of the oral cavity for abnormalities

Complications of Procedure

1. Transient bacteremia causing distant infection
2. Enamel irregularities from improper use of the ultrasonic tooth scaler
3. Inhalation of aerosolized bacteria by the operator
4. Thermal damage to tooth and gingiva

Equipment Needed

1. Examination gloves
2. Cap
3. Mask
4. Cuffed endotracheal tube
5. Equipment necessary for general anesthesia
6. Dental chart (Fig. 25–1)
7. Mouth gag
8. Single-ended or double-ended hand scaling instruments (Fig. 25–2)
9. Dental explorer (Fig. 25–3)
10. Periodontal probe (Fig. 25–4)
11. Ultrasonic tooth scaler or air-turbine scaler and assorted tips (Fig. 25–5)
12. Polishing unit, polishing cups, and polishing compound (Fig. 25–6)
13. 30- or 60-cc syringe and 20-gauge blunted needle
14. Dilute povidone-iodine, 0.2 percent chlorhexidine, or sterile physiologic saline solution

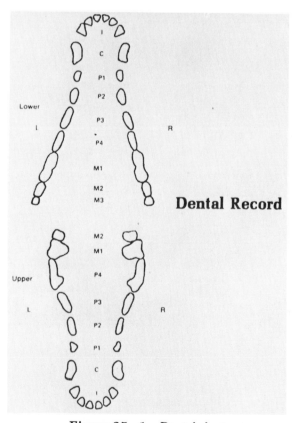

Figure 25–1. Dental chart.

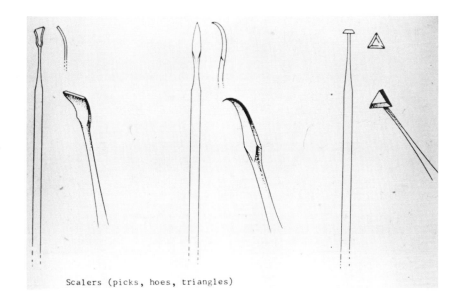

Figure 25-2. Hand scaling instruments.

Scalers (picks, hoes, triangles)

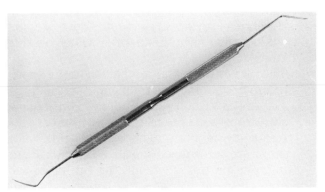

Figure 25-3. Dental explorer.

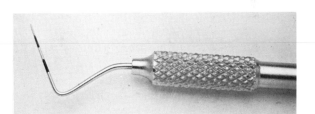

Figure 25-4. Periodontal probe.

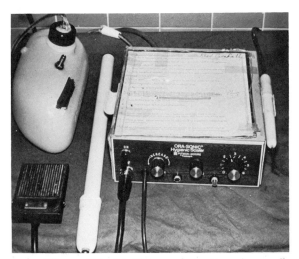

Figure 25-5. Ultrasonic tooth scaler.

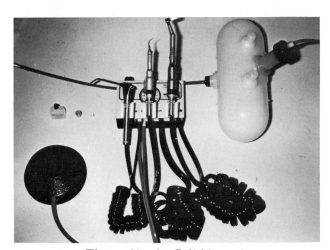

Figure 25-6. Polishing unit.

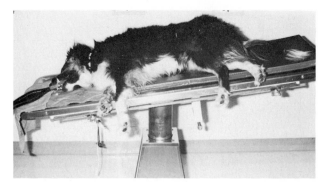

Figure 25–7. Patient on an inclined surface.

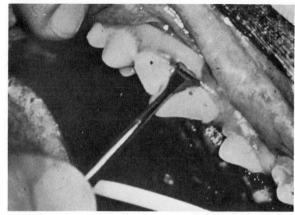

Figure 25–9. Hand scaling tartar from the subgingival space and enamel surface.

Procedure

1. Complete physical examination and pre-anesthetic profile, as the majority of patients are geriatric.
2. Endotracheal intubation (see Chapter 24).
3. The patient is placed in right or left lateral recumbency on an inclined surface with the head tilted down. A grid surface is ideal to allow drainage of fluid and debris (Fig. 25–7).
4. A mouth gag is placed on the canine teeth closest to the table to keep the mouth open.
5. A complete examination of the dental arcade is performed:
   a. *Visual examination:* malocclusions, retained deciduous teeth, loose teeth, cracked teeth, and so forth. Note all abnormalities on the dental chart.
   b. *Instrumentation:* examination of the subgingival region with dental explorer and periodontal pockets with a periodontal probe (Fig. 25–8). Note all abnormalities on the dental chart.
6. Gross tartar accumulations can be removed with hand scaling instruments. The scaler is gently placed in the subgingival space against the enamel surface of the tooth. With pressure against the tooth, the tartar is scaled off (Fig. 25–9).
7. The ultrasonic scaler is adjusted to the appropriate frequency. The frequency is initially set at 0, and the water flow is adjusted until one to two drops per second fall from the tip. The frequency is then adjusted until all water drops are aerosolized. To check adequate tuning, place a finger against the tip for 15 seconds. If no heat is detected, tuning is correct.
8. The ultrasonic scaling tip is moved *lightly* back and forth across the tooth, keeping the tip parallel to the gingival margin (Fig. 25–10). Do not scale a tooth for more than 15

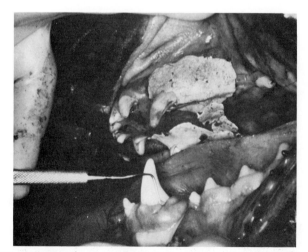

Figure 25–8. Examination of periodontal pocket with a periodontal probe.

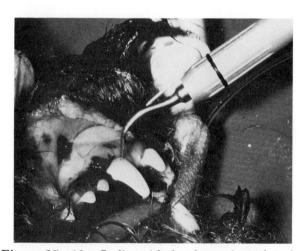

Figure 25–10. Scaling with the ultrasonic tooth scaler.

seconds. Proper scaling requires subgingival tartar removal.

9. First scale the buccal surface of the uppermost teeth, then the lingual surface of the downside teeth. Turn the patient over and repeat the procedures described in Steps 4 through 8.

10. Areas that are difficult to scale ultrasonically (such as crowded teeth, subgingival calculus, periodontal pockets, and so on) should be hand scaled.

11. After scaling is complete, the irregular pitted surfaces of the enamel created by scaling are polished. Polishing compound is mixed into a thin paste and placed in the polishing cup. Polishing is done with firm pressure for a short time (15 seconds). All tooth surfaces are polished (Fig. 25–11).

12. A 30- to 60-cc syringe with a blunt-tipped 20-gauge needle is filled with dilute povidone-iodine, 0.2 percent chlorhexidine, or sterile physiologic saline solution. The gingival sulcus is flushed to remove any traces of dislodged calculus or other debris.

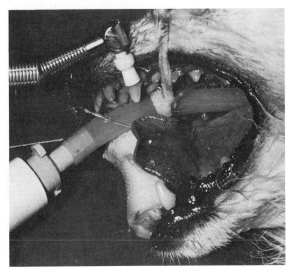

Figure 25–11. Polishing the enamel surface of the tooth.

13. All dental abnormalities, extractions, and treatment regimens are recorded on the patient's dental chart and placed in the permanent record.

SUGGESTED READING

Hawkins JB: Periodontal disease: Therapy and prevention. Vet Clin North Am 16(5):835–850, 1986.

Transtracheal Aspiration

Purpose of Procedure

1. To allow sterile collection of a sample of fluid and/or cells from the trachea

Complications of Procedure

1. Laceration of the tracheal or laryngeal mucosa resulting in hemorrhage or subcutaneous emphysema
2. Pulmonary aspiration of the catheter due to inadvertent cutting of catheter during the procedure
3. Destabilization of a patient due to positioning or stress of the procedure, resulting in respiratory distress
4. Pneumothorax

Equipment Needed

1. Through-the-needle catheter
   Cats and dogs <20 lbs   19-gauge catheter, 8 inches
   Dogs 20 to 50 lbs   19-gauge catheter, 12 inches
   Dogs >50 lbs   16-gauge catheter, 18 inches
2. Clipper and number 40 clipper blade
3. Surgical scrub and alcohol
4. Lidocaine, 0.5 ml in a syringe with a 25-gauge needle
5. Sterile, empty 12-cc syringe
6. Sterile saline, 0.12 ml/kg body weight, in a syringe
7. Sterile surgical gloves
8. Sterile or clean endotracheal tube (cat only)

Preparation for Procedure

1. Sedate or tranquilize patient if needed.
2. Place patient in sternal recumbency on an examination table, with head and neck extended dorsally. Overextension of the neck can result in decreased patient cooperation or increased respiratory distress.
3. Clip an area over the larynx, centered over the cricothyroid ligament.
4. Surgically prepare clipped area.

Procedure — Canine

1. Don surgical gloves.
2. Palpate the larynx and locate the cricothyroid ligament with the index finger. The ligament is located between the thyroid cartilage and the cricoid cartilage and feels like a semisoft indentation on the ventral surface of the larynx (Fig. 26–1).

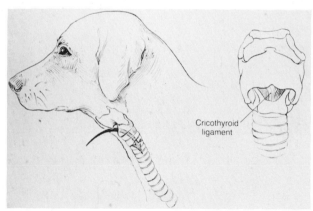

Figure 26–1. Location of cricothyroid ligament. (Courtesy of Dr. S.L. Wheeler.)

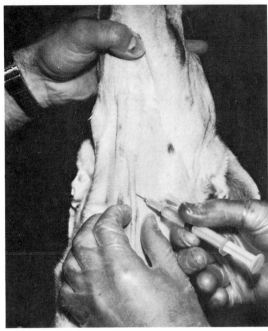

Figure 26–2. Injection of local anesthetic prior to needle insertion. (Courtesy of Dr. S.L. Wheeler.)

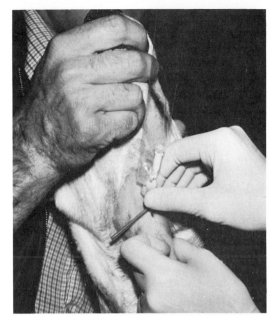

Figure 26–4. Catheter threaded into trachea. (Courtesy of Dr. S.L. Wheeler.)

3. Instill 0.25 to 0.5 ml of lidocaine into the skin and underlying subcutaneous tissue over the ligament (Fig. 26–2).

4. Stabilize the larynx with the free hand.

5. Insert the needle of the catheter bevel down through the cricothyroid ligament and into the trachea. Alternatively, the needle may be placed between the tracheal rings, 1 to 3 cm distal to the larynx. The needle should be pointed at approximately a 135-degree angle from vertical to allow

placement within the trachea and avoid laceration of the dorsal surface of the larynx (Fig. 26–3).

6. Thread the catheter into the trachea, stabilizing the needle with the free hand (Fig. 26–4). In small patients, the catheter tip should be placed approximately three-fourths the distance to the bifurcation of the trachea. In larger patients, the catheter can be threaded to its full length.

7. Withdraw the needle from the larynx and cover it with the provided needle guard (Fig. 26–5).

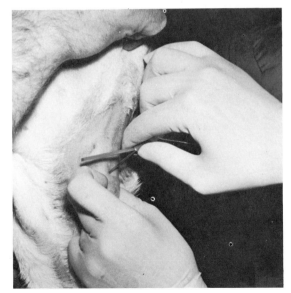

Figure 26–3. Insertion of needle through cricothyroid ligament into trachea. (Courtesy of Dr. S.L. Wheeler.)

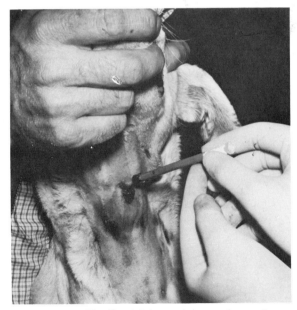

Figure 26–5. Needle withdrawn from trachea and covered with needle guard. (Courtesy of Dr. S.L. Wheeler.)

8. Attach the syringe containing the sterile saline to the catheter adapter and inject half of the premeasured saline at a rapid rate. This will induce coughing in most patients.

9. Quickly disconnect the saline syringe and attach the empty syringe to the catheter.

10. Aspirate repeatedly from the catheter, each time disconnecting the catheter to express most of the air before aspirating again. Care must be taken not to lose the collected contents of the syringe each time (hold the syringe with the tip pointed dorsally). When no further fluid is obtained, repeat Steps 8 to 10 with the remaining saline. Although repeated aspiration after injection increases yield, one can expect to collect only a fraction of the injected saline.

11. Remove the syringe from the catheter.

12. Remove the catheter from the trachea.

13. Submit the collected sample for the desired tests (cytology, culture, and sensitivity).

14. Record the time of the procedure in the patient's record and observe the patient closely for signs of respiratory distress for 1 hour.

Procedure — Feline

1. Obtain a sterile (if possible) or well-cleaned endotracheal tube, 3.0 to 4.0 mm internal diameter.

2. Anesthetize and intubate the patient as described in Chapter 24. Generally the safest method of anesthesia for the respiratory patient is to be placed in a "cat box" and induced using inhalant anesthesia, without the use of injectable agents, thus allowing for rapid and complete recovery. The patient should be kept as lightly anesthetized as possible while still allowing intubation, as a cough reflex is desired when injecting the saline into the trachea.

3. Pass the catheter through the endotracheal tube and into the trachea.

4. Follow Steps 8 to 14 above under *Canine*.

Centesis

BARBARA H. McGUIRE

CYSTOCENTESIS

Purpose of Procedure

1. To obtain a sterile urine sample for urinalysis and/or culture and sensitivity testing
2. To evacuate a bladder that cannot be catheterized. This technique should be used only as a last resort in an animal with urinary obstruction, as laceration of the bladder can result.

Complications of Procedure

1. Hematuria
2. Laceration of the bladder, especially if overdistended
3. Laceration of the bowel, resulting in peritonitis

Equipment Needed

1. 12-cc syringe
2. 1-inch (for small dogs and cats) or 1½-inch (for larger dogs) 22-gauge needle
3. Alcohol and cotton balls

Procedure-Lateral Cystocentesis

1. Place patient on examination table either in lateral recumbency or standing.

2. Palpate bladder to determine size and location.
3. Hold the syringe in the hand nearest the patient's hindquarters and stabilize the bladder from below with the free hand. The bladder should be pressed dorsally and caudally to immobilize it against the pelvis (Fig. 27–1).
4. Wipe area of insertion with alcohol.
5. Insert the needle into the abdominal cavity and bladder, angling caudomedially (Fig. 27–2).
6. Aspirate urine into syringe. If blood is obtained, stop aspiration and withdraw the needle.
7. If no urine is obtained, do not redirect the needle within the abdominal cavity. Withdraw the needle completely, replace the needle, and try again. After two attempts, return the patient to the cage and try again later.

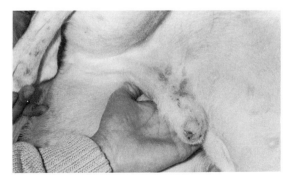

Figure 27–1. Stabilization of bladder, lateral cystocentesis.

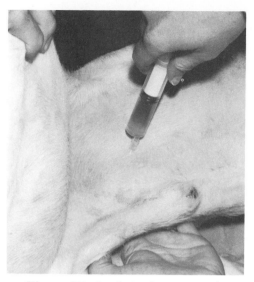

Figure 27–2. Lateral cystocentesis.

Procedure — Ventral Cystocentesis

1. Place the patient in dorsal recumbency. This often requires two assistants for larger dogs, as keeping the patient straight is important to the success of the procedure.

2. Drip alcohol onto the caudal abdomen. The place where the alcohol pools is where the needle should be inserted. If this is not possible, stabilize the bladder against the pelvis with one hand as described above.

3. Insert the needle into the abdomen, staying on the midline (Fig. 27–3).

4. Complete Steps 6 and 7 of *Lateral Cystocentesis.*

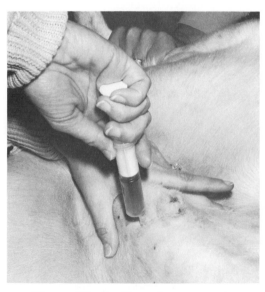

Figure 27–3. Ventral cystocentesis.

Note: Although cystocentesis is a routine procedure, it is also invasive and should not be performed casually. Do not attempt repeated cystocenteses without considering the potential risks to the patient.

ABDOMINOCENTESIS

Purpose of Procedure

1. To obtain a sample of fluid when peritoneal effusion is present
2. To investigate for the presence of fluid if there is suspicion of effusion

Complications of Procedure

1. Laceration of intestine resulting in peritonitis
2. Laceration of spleen resulting in hemoperitoneum

Equipment Needed

1. 1-inch 22-gauge needle
2. Intravenous extension tubing
3. 6-cc syringe
4. Surgical scrub, alcohol, and cotton balls
5. Clippers and number 40 blade
6. Sterile surgical gloves

Preparation for Procedure

1. Attach the extension tubing to the syringe on one end and the needle on the other. By placing a length of tubing between the needle and syringe, sudden movements by the patient will result in less trauma by the needle than when the needle is directly attached to the syringe. The needle is able to move freely with the patient.

2. Place the patient on an examination table in right lateral recumbency.

3. Clip and surgically prepare an area on the abdomen extending from the midline dorsally 4 to 6 cm and from the umbilicus caudally 4 to 6 cm.

4. Don the surgical gloves.

Procedure

1. Repeat the following procedure in four locations as shown in Figure 27–4. Two of the locations

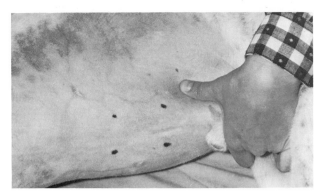

Figure 27-4. Points of needle insertion for four-quadrant abdominocentesis.

should be located on the midline (cranially and caudally) and two 3 to 5 cm dorsal to the midline (cranially and caudally).

2. Insert the needle into the abdominal cavity at a slow rate, continually aspirating during insertion (Fig. 27-5). The needle should be directed perpendicular to the skin. When fluid is obtained in the hub of the needle, discontinue needle insertion and hold the needle at that depth. If no fluid is obtained, rotation of the needle or gentle redirection within the abdomen can be helpful.

3. Continue to aspirate fluid until the flow stops or adequate fluid is obtained.

4. Submit the fluid for cytology and culture and sensitivity testing as desired.

5. If no fluid is obtained, repeat the procedure in each of the four locations until fluid is obtained.

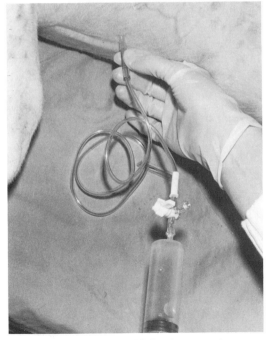

Figure 27-5. Abdominocentesis.

THORACENTESIS

Purpose of Procedure

1. To obtain a sample of fluid for diagnostic purposes in cases of suspected pleural effusion

2. To evacuate the thoracic cavity in cases of pleural effusion, hydrothorax, or pneumothorax, thus relieving respiratory distress

Complications of Procedure

1. Pulmonary laceration resulting in pleural or pulmonary hemorrhage

2. Pulmonary laceration resulting in pneumothorax

3. Myocardial puncture resulting in hemorrhage or arrhythmia

Equipment Needed

1. Canine—1-inch 20- or 22-gauge needle attached to an intravenous extension tube
    Feline—23-gauge "butterfly" catheter

2. Three-way stopcock

3. 12-, 20-, or 60-cc syringe, depending on the volume of fluid or air to be evacuated. If a large volume is suspected, use a large syringe.

4. Sterile surgical gloves

5. Surgical scrub and alcohol, cotton balls

6. Clippers and number 40 blade

7. Collection bowl (for pleural effusion or hydrothorax)

Preparation for Procedure

1. Extreme care must be taken with the patient with pleural effusion or pneumothorax, as further respiratory distress may occur owing to manipulation or positioning. Sternal recumbency is often the most comfortable position for these patients and should be used if the patient resists being placed in lateral recumbency.

2. Local anesthesia is not necessary, and tranquilization is often contraindicated in these patients owing to respiratory depression; therefore, good assistance and restraint are needed.

3. After placement in sternal recumbency, widely clip the lateral thorax, concentrating on the ventrolateral area if fluid is suspected and the dorsolateral area if air is suspected.

4. Surgically prepare the clipped area of the thorax.

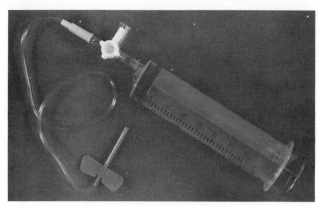

Figure 27–6. Aspiration assembly for thoracentesis.

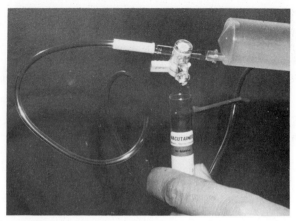

Figure 27–8. Expression of fluid from three-way stopcock into glass tube.

5.   Attach the needle and tubing or the butterfly catheter to the three-way stopcock and then to the syringe (Fig. 27–6).

6.   Don the surgical gloves.

Procedure

1.   The preferred entry point for thoracentesis is the seventh or eighth intercostal space. If pneumothorax is suspected, needle placement should be dorsolateral. If pleural effusion is suspected, placement should be ventrolateral (Fig. 27–7).

2.   Check the stopcock to be sure it is open to the patient (outflow closed).

3.   Insert the needle into the thorax along the cranial surface of the rib. The intercostal vessels and nerves are located caudal to each rib and should be avoided. During insertion, aspirate with the syringe to create negative pressure. As soon as fluid or air is obtained, stop insertion and hold the needle at that point. The butterfly catheter used in cats can

be released during the remaining procedure and it will stay in place. If a hypodermic needle and tubing are used, the needle must be held in place throughout the procedure, thus requiring an assistant to manipulate the stopcock.

4.   When the syringe is full, close the stopcock to the patient and express the air or fluid from the syringe. If fluid is obtained, place a sample in the appropriate collection tubes for analysis (Fig. 27–8), collecting the rest in the collection bowl.

5.   Repeat the aspiration and ejection until no further fluid or air is obtained. Count the number of times the syringe is emptied to calculate total volume removed.

6.   If pneumothorax is present, more air can often be obtained by changing to lateral recumbency. The patient usually tolerates this position once the majority of the air is removed.

7.   Record the total volume of fluid or air obtained in the patient's record and submit the fluid for laboratory analysis.

PERICARDIOCENTESIS

Purpose of Procedure

1.   To obtain a sample of pericardial fluid for cytologic evaluation

2.   To remove pericardial fluid to relieve cardiac tamponade

Complications of Procedure

1.   Pulmonary laceration resulting in hemorrhage or pneumothorax

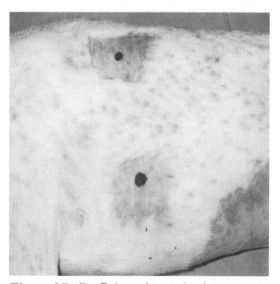

Figure 27–7. Points of entry for thoracentesis.

Figure 27–9. Catheter prepared for pericardiocentesis.

2. Myocardial laceration resulting in hemorrhage or arrhythmias

Equipment Needed

1. 14- or 16-gauge 5½-inch over-the-needle radiopaque catheter with three sideholes cut near the tip (Fig. 27–9)
2. Number 15 scalpel blade
3. 1 ml lidocaine in a 3-cc syringe, 25-gauge needle
4. Empty 3-cc syringe
5. Three-way stopcock attached to a 20-cc syringe
6. EKG machine
7. Surgical scrub and alcohol, cotton balls
8. Sterile surgical gloves
9. Clippers and number 40 blade

Preparation for Procedure

1. Attach EKG lead to the patient in the standard manner. The EKG should be monitored continually during the procedure to detect ventricular arrhythmias, an indication of myocardial contact with the needle.
2. The procedure can be performed with the patient standing or in left lateral recumbency.
3. Palpate the thorax for maximum cardiac impulse. Clip an area of the right fourth to sixth intercostal spaces over the cardiac impulse.
4. Surgically prepare clipped skin.
5. Don sterile gloves.
6. Attach empty 3-cc syringe to the catheter needle hub.

Procedure

1. Locally infiltrate an area just lateral to the sternum and cranial to the fifth or sixth rib (Fig. 27–10).

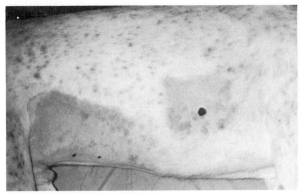

Figure 27–10. Point of insertion for pericardiocentesis.

2. Make a stab incision in the skin with the scalpel blade.
3. Insert the needle (with catheter) through the incision and slowly advance it toward the heart. Apply mild suction to the syringe during advancement.
4. When fluid is obtained, advance the catheter over the needle into the pericardial sac.
5. Withdraw the needle and attach the three-way stopcock and 20-cc syringe to the adapter of the catheter.
6. With the stopcock open to the patient, aspirate fluid from the pericardial sac.
7. Close the stopcock to the patient and express the fluid into appropriate containers for evaluation.
8. Repeat Steps 6 and 7 until no further fluid is obtained. The patient's position can be changed to allow more complete drainage.
9. Record the volume of fluid obtained in the patient's record and submit the fluid for examination.

Notes

1. If arrhythmias are seen on the EKG during pericardiocentesis, it indicates myocardial contact. Withdrawal of the needle usually results in conversion to a normal rhythm.
2. If the fluid obtained resembles peripheral blood, compare the fluid to a sample of peripheral blood. Pericardial fluid usually does not clot and has a packed cell volume different from that of peripheral blood.

ADDITIONAL READING

Thomas WP: Pericardial disease. *In* Ettinger SJ (ed): Textbook of Veterinary Internal Medicine. Philadelphia, WB Saunders, 1983.

CHAPTER

28

BARBARA McGUIRE

Cerebrospinal Fluid Collection

Purpose of Procedure

1. To obtain a sample of cerebrospinal fluid (CSF) for laboratory examination
2. To allow measurement of CSF pressure
3. To allow access to the subarachnoid space for radiographic study (myelography)

Complications of Procedure

1. Unsuccessful collection
2. Hemorrhage into CSF due to puncture of vertebral sinuses
3. Herniation of the brain resulting in respiratory or cardiac dysfunction or arrest. CSF collection should not be performed on patients that are suspected of having very high CSF pressures or that are at risk for herniation
4. Puncture of the medulla due to incorrect placement of the spinal needle during CSF tap
5. Infection of CNS due to lack of asepsis during procedures

Note: Serious complications of a CSF collection do occur but are rare if proper technique is used and careful consideration is given to the condition of the patient.

Equipment Needed

1. 20-gauge (large dogs) or 22-gauge (smaller dogs and cats) 1½-inch spinal needle with stylet for cisternal puncture of 2½-inch (same gauge) spinal needle with stylet for lumbar puncture
2. Sterile glass tubes for collection of fluid
3. Manometer with three-way stopcock (stopcock outflow closed)

4. Sterile surgical gloves
5. Sterile surgical drape, 3-inch aperture
6. Surgical scrub, alcohol, and cotton balls
7. Clippers and number 40 blade

CISTERNAL PUNCTURE

Preparation for Procedure

1. The patient should be placed under general anesthesia, as complete immobilization is required for this procedure.
2. Place the patient in lateral recumbency—right lateral recumbency for right-handed individuals and left lateral recumbency for left-handed individuals.
3. Clip the dorsal surface of the cranial cervical spine, extending above the external occipital protuberance and below the wings of the atlas.
4. Surgically prepare the entire clipped area.
5. Position the patient so that the cervical spine is placed at the edge of the table. Flex the head ventrally and lift the nose slightly to keep the spine straight and the head at a 90-degree angle to the axis of the cervical spine (Fig. 28–1).
6. Drape the cervical region, with the drape aperture centered over the clipped area.

Procedure

Note: the following figures are shown without a drape for better visualization.

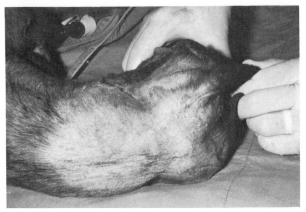

Figure 28–1. Proper positioning for cisternal puncture.

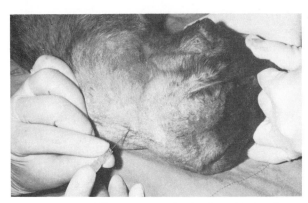

Figure 28–3. Advancement of spinal needle for cisternal tap.

1. The location for puncture can be found by imagining two lines, one drawn vertically across the neck between the cranial borders of the wings of the atlas and the other running caudally from the external occipital protuberance (Fig. 28–2). The point of entry is located where these lines intersect.

2. Insert the needle, bevel toward the patient's head, through the skin and advance it toward the spinal canal, keeping it at a right angle to the spine. During advancement, stabilize the needle with the free hand, which should be placed against the patient (Fig. 28–3). This allows the needle to move with the patient if there is any unexpected motion.

3. During advancement, periodically remove the stylet to check for CSF appearance, always stabilizing the hub of the needle with the free hand (Fig. 28–4). If pure blood is obtained, withdraw the needle and start over with a fresh needle. If bone is contacted with the needle, carefully "walk" the needle cranially or caudally to enter the atlanto-occipi-

tal space. *Note:* If high CSF pressure is detected by a very rapid flow of CSF from the needle, immediately withdraw the needle from the patient to prevent rapid herniation of the brain due to excessive or rapid fluid removal.

4. When fluid is obtained, carefully attach the manometer to the needle and allow the manometer to fill until the level remains stable.

5. Record the CSF pressure, then close the stopcock to the needle and collect the fluid for analysis. The fluid should be allowed to drip into the collection tubes, as aspiration with a syringe can result in hemorrhage. When the manometer empties, remove the manometer from the needle and replace the stylet.

6. Remove the needle from the patient and recover the patient from anesthesia, observing respiratory and cardiovascular function carefully to detect brain stem herniation.

7. Submit the collected cerebrospinal fluid for analysis.

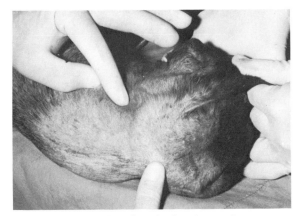

Figure 28–2. Landmarks for cisternal puncture.

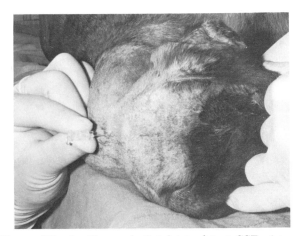

Figure 28–4. Removal of stylet to detect CSF, cisternal puncture.

Cerebrospinal Fluid Collection **187**

Preparation for Procedure

1. The patient should be placed under general anesthesia.
2. Place the patient in lateral recumbency— right lateral recumbency for right-handed individuals and left lateral recumbency for left-handed individuals. The lumbar spine should be placed along the edge of the table.
3. Widely clip and surgically prepare the dorsal lumbosacral spine.
4. Flex the lumbar spine by having the assistant bring the front and hind legs together.
5. Don surgical gloves.

Procedure

1. Palpate the dorsal processes of the lumbar spine and identify the L6—L7 space (Fig. 28–5).
2. The needle is inserted perpendicular to the

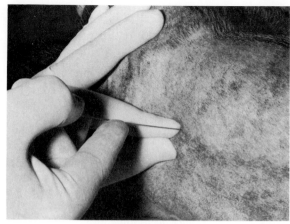

Figure 28–6. Insertion of needle for lumbar puncture. Note that insertion is lateral to the dorsal process (fingers placed on processes).

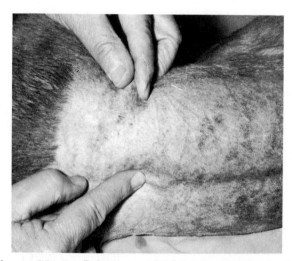

Figure 28–5. Palpation of L6-L7 interspace for lumbar puncture.

spine just lateral and cranial to the dorsal process of L7 and directed toward the midline (Fig. 28–6). When the bone is encountered, "walk" the tip of the needle cranially or caudally until it enters the intervetebral space. Penetration of the interarcuate ligament can often be felt, and the patient may flinch as the needle penetrates the dura.

3. Remove the stylet and check for the presence of CSF. If no flow is seen, continue to advance the needle, periodically checking for flow. If bone is again encountered, the ventral canal of the spinal column has been met. Withdraw the needle slightly and remove the stylet to see if fluid can be collected from the ventral subarachnoid space.
4. When fluid is obtained, allow it to drip into collection tubes. CSF flow from a lumbar puncture is much slower than from a cisternal puncture.
5. Replace the stylet and withdraw the needle from the patient.
6. If no fluid is obtained, attempts can be made at the L5—L6 or L4—L5 space.
7. Recover the patient from anesthesia, carefully monitoring cardiovascular and respiratory function.

ADDITIONAL READING

Greene CE, Oliver JE: Neurologic examination. *In* Ettinger SJ (ed): Textbook of Veterinary Internal Medicine, Vol 1. Philadelphia, WB Saunders, 1983.
Oliver JE, Lorenz MD: Handbook of Veterinary Neurologic Diagnosis. Philadelphia, WB Saunders, 1983.

Peritoneal Catheterization and Lavage

PERITONEAL CATHETERIZATION

Purpose of Procedure

1. As a diagnostic aid, in conjunction with peritoneal lavage, to improve retrieval of a peritoneal sample
2. As a therapeutic aid, to remove excess fluid from the peritoneal cavity or in preparation for peritoneal lavage

Complications of Procedure

1. Rupture of an abdominal viscus leading to hemorrhage, infection, or inflammation
2. Infection
3. Hemorrhage
4. Subcutaneous leakage of fluid
5. Catheter plugging

Equipment Needed

1. Sterile gloves
2. Clipper and number 40 blade
3. Surgical scrub and alcohol, cotton balls
4. Peritoneal catheter set or 14- to 16-gauge over-the-needle type catheter (Fig. 29–1)
5. 2 percent lidocaine
6. Number 10 and 11 scalpel blades
7. Sterile drapes
8. Extension tubing
9. Three-way stopcock
10. Syringes
11. Tubes for sample collection

Procedure

1. Evacuate the urinary bladder.
2. Restrain the patient in lateral recumbency.
3. Clip the hair from a rectangular area surrounding the umbilicus.
4. Surgically prepare the skin.
5. Don sterile gloves.
6. Infiltrate a 1-cm area 1 cm caudal to the umbilicus with 1.0 ml 2 percent lidocaine.
7. With the number 10 scalpel blade, make four or five holes in the distal end of the catheter, being careful not to cut out more than 90 degrees from the circumference of the catheter (Fig. 29–2).
8. Make a 5-mm stab incision with the number 11 scalpel blade through the skin in the center of the locally anesthetized area.
9. Using a controlled push, drive trocar and catheter through subcutis, linea alba/abdominal muscles, and peritoneum.
10. Direct the apparatus dorsocaudally and advance the catheter while holding the trocar in place.

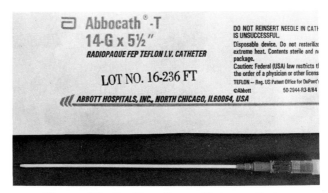

Figure 29–1. Over-the-needle type catheter.

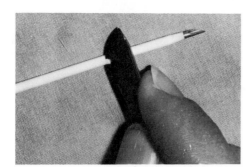

Figure 29 – 2. Additional holes are made in the distal end of the catheter.

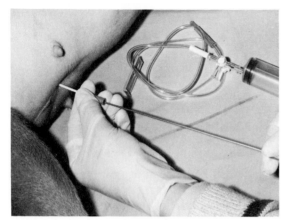

Figure 29 – 3. The trocar is retracted from the catheter.

11. Retract the trocar and attach the extension tubing and three-way stopcock (Fig. 29 – 3).

12. Collect samples by free flow of fluid into tubes or by applying gentle negative pressure with a syringe.

PERITONEAL LAVAGE

Purpose of Procedure

1. As a diagnostic aid, to determine the presence of a localized peritonitis

2. As a therapeutic aid, to dialyze a patient with severe renal failure or as an adjunct in the treatment of peritonitis

Complications of Procedure

1. Same as those mentioned above and, in addition, causing a localized peritonitis to become generalized

Equipment Needed

1. As above
2. Suture material, needle holders, and scissors
3. Bandage material
4. Antibacterial ointment
5. Warm balanced electrolyte solution or dialysate

Procedure

1. Place peritoneal catheter as above. Connect sterile extension tubing and three-way stopcock.

2. Make a tape butterfly (see Fig. 21 – 11) on the exposed end of the catheter and suture the peritoneal catheter to the skin with mattress sutures (see Fig. 21 – 13).

3. Apply a small amount of antibacterial ointment to the skin at the point of catheter entry.

4. Immobilize the catheter by bandaging the entire abdomen with gauze and tape such that only the three-way stopcock is visible (Fig. 29 – 4).

5. Instill 20 ml of warm balanced electrolyte solution or dialysate per kilogram of body weight into the peritoneal cavity by gravity flow.

6. Roll the patient gently from side to side.

7. The infused fluid is siphoned by gravity flow into the original container by placing this container lower than the patient.

8. Aliquots of fluid can be removed via the three-way stopcock for cytologic (EDTA tube) and microbiologic (clot tube) analysis.

9. If the fluid was placed for dialysis, it should be left in place for 30 to 45 minutes before removing to allow equilibration.

10. If the catheter is to be left in place, flush with heparinized saline every 4 hours and change bandage daily or more frequently, if necessary.

11. Replace the catheter every 48 to 72 hours.

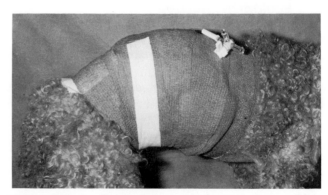

Figure 29 – 4. The catheter is bandaged in place with the three-way stopcock exposed.

RECOMMENDED READING

1. Crane SW: Diagnostic peritoneal lavage. *In* Kirk RW: Current Veterinary Therapy. Philadelphia, WB Saunders, 1986, p 3.
2. Ettinger SJ: Ascites, peritonitis, and other causes of abdominal enlargement. *In* Textbook of Veterinary Internal Medicine. Philadelphia, WB Saunders, 1989, p 132.

CHAPTER

30

BARBARA H. McGUIRE

Bone Marrow Aspiration

Purpose of Procedure

1. To obtain a diagnostic sample of bone marrow cells when clinically indicated
2. To gain access to the marrow cavity for therapeutic purposes, e.g., blood transfusion or fluid therapy in neonatal and very small patients

Complications of Procedure

1. Subcutaneous or dermal hemorrhage
2. Iatrogenic injury to underlying muscles or nerves

Equipment Needed

1. Bone marrow aspiration needle
    16-gauge Rosenthal needle for large dogs
    18-gauge Rosenthal needle for small dogs and cats
2. Sterile 12-cc syringe
3. Number 15 scalpel blade
4. 2 percent lidocaine in a 3-cc syringe, 25-gauge needle
5. Sterile surgical drape
6. Surgical scrub and alcohol, cotton balls
7. Precleaned microscope slides
8. Sterile surgical gloves
9. 3-0 nylon suture, cutting needle

Procedure — Iliac Crest Aspiration

1. Place the patient in sternal or lateral recumbency, with the side to be aspirated upward. Mild sedation may be necessary in fractious patients.

2. Clip and surgically prepare a 7- to 8-cm square centered over the iliac crest.
3. Place the sterile drape over the clipped area and don the surgical gloves.
4. Locate the point of intended needle entry and infiltrate the skin, subcutaneous tissue, and periosteum with the 2 percent lidocaine. The entry point should be located at the widest portion of the dorsal border of the iliac crest (Fig. 30–1).
5. Make a small 2- to 3-mm stab incision with the scalpel blade at the point of entry.
6. With the stylet in place, introduce the needle into the incision and advance it through the subcutaneous tissue to the bone of the crest.
7. When bone is encountered, center the needle over the widest part of the iliac crest and begin careful introduction into the bone. Advance the needle into the middle of the crest, aiming slightly

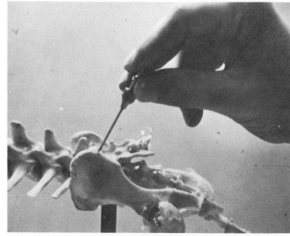

Figure 30–1. Point of needle insertion, iliac crest (located at the widest portion of the dorsal border of the iliac crest).

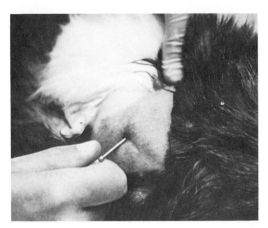

Figure 30–2. Direction of needle advancement into the iliac crest. (The hub of the needle is slightly caudal and lateral to a vertical line through the iliac crest.)

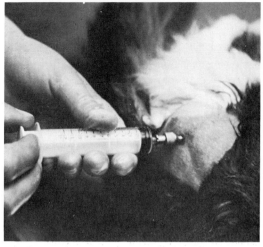

Figure 30–4. Negative pressure for aspiration, iliac crest (negative pressure applied to syringe).

caudal to a vertical line through the iliac crest (Fig. 30–2). Slowly rotate the needle until it is firmly embedded in the bone (Fig. 30–3).

8.   Remove the stylet from the needle and attach the 12-cc syringe.

9.   Apply brisk negative pressure on the syringe (Fig. 30–4). When blood appears in the needle hub, immediately release the negative pressure to avoid contamination with excess peripheral blood.

10.   Quickly disconnect the syringe from the needle and place a drop of the aspirated material on three or four of the prepared microscope slides. Immediately make a pull slide preparation with each slide (see Chapter 18). Speed is essential to prevent coagulation of the sample prior to slide preparation.

11.   When an adequate sample is obtained, replace the stylet and withdraw the needle from the crest.

12.   Apply digital pressure with a gauze sponge over the aspiration site for 3 to 5 minutes to prevent hemorrhage. This is especially important in patients with coagulopathies.

13.   Close the skin incision with a cruciate suture using the nylon suture material.

Procedure — Trochanteric Fossa Aspiration

1.   Place the patient in lateral recumbency on an examination table.

2.   Clip and surgically prepare a 7- to 8-cm area centered over the greater trochanter.

3.   Place the drape over the prepared area and don surgical gloves.

4.   Locate the trochanteric fossa by palpation of the greater trochanter. The fossa is located just me-

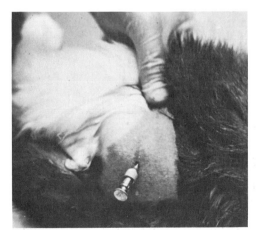

Figure 30–3. Bone marrow needle firmly embedded within bone.

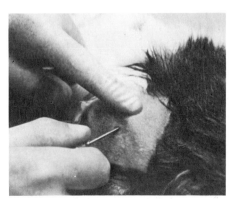

Figure 30–5. Palpation of greater trochanter for location of fossa.

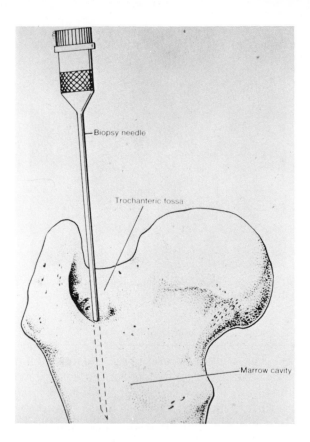

Biopsy needle

Trochanteric fossa

Marrow cavity

Figure 30–6. Direction of needle for trochanteric fossa aspiration (parallel to shaft of femur and medial to trochanteric fossa).

dial to the trochanter (Fig. 30–5). Locally infiltrate the skin, subcutaneous tissue, and periosteum using the 2 percent lidocaine.

5. Make a 2- to 3-cm stab incision in the skin over the trochanteric fossa.

6. Introduce the needle into the incision and carefully advance it through the soft tissue until

bone is encountered. The direction of the needle should be parallel to the shaft of the femur to allow placement within the marrow cavity (Fig. 30–6).

7. Slowly rotate the needle until it is firmly embedded within the marrow cavity.

8. Complete Steps 8 to 13 as described for Iliac Crest Aspiration.

APPENDICES

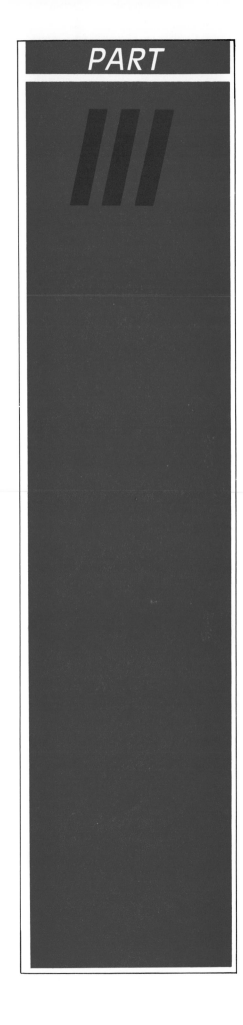

PART

III

Sample Requirements for Laboratory Tests

TEST DESCRIPTION	SPECIMEN
These recommendations are only guidelines. Sample requirements may vary depending on each laboratory's protocol. Consult your own laboratory for specific instructions.	
Acid-base balance	3 ml heparinized whole blood (arterial sample preferred)
ACTH (adrenocorticotropic hormone)	12 ml plasma; frozen—separate into two 6-ml vials
A/G ratio (total protein, albumin, A/G)	2 ml serum
ALA (aminoelevulinic acid)	20-ml aliquot of 24-hr urine Add 6N HCl to pH 1–2. Note 24-hr volume.
Albumin	2 ml serum
Alkaline phosphatase	1 ml serum
Alkaline phosphatase isoenzymes	2 ml serum frozen
Ammonia, blood	3 ml heparinized plasma; freeze immediately
Amylase, fluid	1 ml fluid
Amylase, serum	1 ml serum
Amylase, urine	10 ml random urine
ANA (anti-nuclear antibody)	2 ml serum
Bence Jones protein	30 ml fresh random urine
Bile, urine, qualitative	2 ml random urine
Bilirubin, direct	1 ml serum (do not expose to light)
Bilirubin, total	1 ml serum (do not expose to light)
Bilirubin, urine, qualitative	5 ml random urine
Brucella titer, canine	1 ml serum
BSP (bromsulphalein)	3 ml EDTA-plasma
Buffy coat preparation	EDTA tube
BUN (blood urea nitrogen)	1 ml serum
Calcium, serum	2 ml serum
Calcium, serum, ionized	3 ml serum
Calcium, urine	25-ml aliquot of 24-hr urine. Add 6N HCl to pH 1–2. Note 24-hr volume.
Carbon dioxide content (CO$_2$)	2 ml serum
Carbon monoxide (carboxyhemoglobin)	1 gray top
Chloride, CSF	1 ml CSF
Chloride, fluid	1 ml fluid
Chloride, serum	1 ml serum
Chloride, urine	24-ml aliquot of 24-hr urine. Note 24-hr volume.
Cholesterol by enzymatic method	1 ml serum
Cholinesterase, RBC	2 ml heparinized blood
Cholinesterase, serum	1 ml serum
CK isoenzymes	1 ml serum
Coagulation factors	
Activated partial thromboplastin time (APTT)	Plasma, frozen. Two 1-ml aliquots—blue top
Factor VIII	Plasma, frozen. Two 1-ml aliquots—blue top

Table continued on following page

TEST DESCRIPTION	SPECIMEN
Factor IX	Plasma, frozen. Two 1-ml aliquots — blue top
Factor XI	Plasma, frozen. Two 1-ml aliquots — blue top
Factor XII	Plasma, frozen. Two 1-ml aliquots — blue top
Factor XIII	Plasma, frozen. Two 1-ml aliquots — blue top
Fibrin split products	Plasma, 2 ml. Collect in special blue-top vial containing thrombin and special enzyme inhibitor.
Fibrin stabilizing factor (factor XIII)	Plasma, frozen. Two 1-ml aliquots — blue top
Fibrinogen titer	Plasma, frozen. Two 1-ml aliquots — blue top
Partial thromboplastin time (see APTT)	Plasma, frozen. Two 1-ml aliquots — blue top
Plasma clot lysis	Plasma, frozen. Two 1-ml aliquots — blue top
Platelet count	EDTA tube
Platelet factor 3	1-ml plasma; need not be frozen. Results not valid if there is any clotting of sample or if corticosteroids are given prior to sample drawing — blue top
Prothrombin consumption time	1 ml serum, frozen. Two 1-ml aliquots
Prothrombin time	Plasma, frozen. Two 1-ml aliquots — blue top
Russell's viper venom time	Plasma, frozen. Two 1-ml aliquots — blue top
Coccidioidomycosis antibody, screening	2 ml serum
Cold agglutinins	2 ml serum
Coombs, direct	1 red top
canine or feline	
Coombs, indirect	1 red top
canine or feline	
Copper, serum	2 ml serum
Copper, urine	100-ml aliquot of 24-hr urine. Note 24-hr volume.
Cortisol, serum or plasma	3 ml serum or heparinized plasma
Cortisol, urine	10-ml aliquot of 24-hr urine frozen. Note 24-hr volume.
Creatine kinase (CK)	2 ml serum
Creatinine, serum	2 ml serum frozen
Creatinine, urine	10-ml aliquot of 24-hr urine frozen. Note 24-hr volume.
Creatinine clearance	2 ml serum/10-ml aliquot of specifically timed (12 or 24 hr) urine. Note total volume/time.
Cryoglobulins, qualitative	1 red top
11-Deoxy cortisol (compound S)	3 ml heparinized plasma; separate immediately
11-Deoxy/11-Oxy ratio of 17-ketogenic steroids	100-ml aliquot of 24-hr urine. Note 24-hr volume.
Digitoxin, RIA	2 ml serum
Digoxin, RIA	2 ml serum
Dirofilariasis	EDTA tube
D-Xylose tolerance	100-ml aliquot of 5-hr urine. Note total volume.
Electrolytes	2 ml serum
(includes sodium, potassium, chloride, carbon dioxide)	
Electrophoresis, CSF	1 ml CSF
Electrophoresis, hemoglobin	EDTA tube
Electrophoresis, protein, serum	1 ml serum
Electrophoresis, protein, urine	20-ml aliquot of 24-hr urine. Note 24-hr volume.

TEST DESCRIPTION	SPECIMEN
Eosinophil count, direct	EDTA tube
Erythropoietin, quantitative	2 ml serum
ESR (erythrocyte sedimentation rate)	EDTA tube
Estradiol, serum, RIA	5 ml heparinized plasma or serum, frozen
Fatty acids, free	4 ml serum
Feline leukemia virus	3 thin blood smears
Fibrinogen, quantitative	1 blue top
FIP, fluid exam	3 ml fluid in EDTA tube, fixed smear of sediment
Gamma globulins, quantitative (immunoglobulins) (includes IgG, IgA, and IgM)	1 ml serum
GGTP (gamma glutamyl transpeptidase)	1 ml serum
Glucose, blood, fasting	1 gray top
Glucose, CSF	1 ml CSF
Glucose, fluid	1 gray top
Glucose, urine, quantitative	25-ml aliquot of 24-hr urine. Add 250 mg NaF to aliquot and mix. Note 24-hr volume.
Glucose tolerance (3 tests)	3 gray tops (indicate time)
Each Additional Glucose	1 gray top (indicate time)
Heavy metal screen (includes antimony, arsenic, mercury, and bismuth)	50 ml random urine
Hemoglobin, free, urine	10 ml random urine
Hemoglobin electrophoresis	EDTA tube
Hemogram (includes WBC, RBC, Hgb, Hct, MCV, MCH, and MCHC)	EDTA tube
Histoplasmosis, serological screen only	1 red top
Immunoelectrophoresis	1 ml serum. Avoid hemolysis.
Immunoglobulins, quantitative (includes IgG, IgA, and IgM in most species)	1 ml serum
Insulin, plasma	2 ml serum or plasma frozen
Iron, total, and iron-binding capacity	4 ml serum
Lactic acid	Mix 4 ml blood from gray top with 4 ml 7% perchloric acid. (Remove tourniquet before blood withdrawal.)
LDH (Lactic acid dehydrogenase), serum	1 ml serum (Do not freeze.)
LDH isoenzyme pattern	1 ml serum (Do not freeze.)
LE prep	1 red top (Do not mail.)
Lead, blood	1 green top
Lead, urine	100-ml aliquot of 24-hr urine. Note 24-hr volume.
Leptospira agglutinins	2 ml serum
Lipase	2 ml serum
Lipase, total, serum	2 ml serum
Magnesium, serum	1 ml serum
Methemalbumin (Schumm test)	2 ml serum
Methemoglobin	1 gray top, deliver immediately
Microfilaria	EDTA tube
Mucopolysaccharides, qualitative	30 ml random urine
Ornithine carbamyl transferase (OCT)	3 ml serum
Osmolality, serum	2 ml serum
Osmolality, urine	2 ml urine
Oxalate	50-ml aliquot of 24-hr urine. Note 24-hr volume.
Parathyroid hormone (PTH)	8 ml serum frozen

Table continued on following page

TEST DESCRIPTION	SPECIMEN
Phosphatase, alkaline	1 ml serum
Phospholipids	2 ml serum
Phosphorus, serum	1 ml serum
Phosphorus, urine	25-ml aliquot of 24-hr urine. Note 24-hr volume.
Plasma clot lysis	Plasma frozen. Two 1-ml aliquots.
Platelet factor 3	1 lavender or blue. Sample must be free of any clot formation.
Potassium, fluid	1 ml fluid
Potassium, serum	1 ml serum
Potassium, urine	10-ml aliquot of 24-hr urine. Note 24-hr volume.
Protein, total, CSF	2 ml CSF
Protein, total, urine	100-ml aliquot of 24-hr urine. Note 24-hr volume.
Protein, total, serum	1 ml serum
Protein electrophoresis, serum	1 ml serum
Protein electrophoresis, urine	20 ml random urine
Reticulocyte count	EDTA tube
Rheumatoid factor, canine	1 ml serum
Salicylates	1 ml serum
Sedimentation rate (ESR)	EDTA tube
SGOT (transaminase-SGO)	1 ml serum
SGPT (transaminase-SGP)	1 ml serum
Sodium, fluid	1 ml fluid
Sodium, serum	1 ml serum
Sodium, urine	10-ml aliquot of 24-hr urine. Note 24-hr volume.
Specific gravity, fluid	1 ml fluid
T_3 uptake (resin)	1 ml serum
T_4 by RIA	2 ml serum
Free T_4 by equilibrium dialysis	3 ml serum
Testosterone, serum (RIA)	2 ml serum
Testosterone, urine (RIA)	25-ml aliquot of 24-hr urine. Refrigerate sample. Note 24-hr volume.
Thrombin time	Plasma, frozen. Two 1-ml aliquots
Total protein, serum	1 ml serum
Toxoplasma, fluorescent antibody	1 ml serum
Transaminase-SGO	1 ml serum
Transaminase-SGP	1 ml serum
Triglycerides	3 ml serum
Urea nitrogen, blood (BUN)	1 ml serum
Urea nitrogen, urine	10-ml aliquot of 24-hr urine. Note 24-hr volume.
Uric acid, serum	1 ml serum
Uric acid, urine	25-ml aliquot of 24-hr urine. Note 24-hr volume.
Viscosity, serum	6 ml serum
Xylose tolerance	100-ml aliquot of 5-hr urine. Plus 250 mg NaF. Note 5-hr volume.
Zinc, serum	5 ml serum

(From Kirk RW, Bistner SI, Ford R: Handbook of Veterinary Procedures and Emergency Treatment, 5th ed. Philadelphia, W.B. Saunders Co., 1990, pp. 874–879.)

Normal Blood Values*

ERYTHROCYTES	ADULT DOG	AVERAGE	ADULT CAT	AVERAGE
Erythrocytes (millions/μl)	5.5–8.5	6.8	5.5–10.0	7.5
Hemoglobin (gm/dl)	12.0–18.0	14.9	8.0–14.0	12.0
Packed cell volume (vol. %)	37.0–55.0	45.5	24.0–45.0	37.0
Mean corpuscular volume (femtoliters)	66.0–77.0	69.8	40.0–55.0	45.0
Mean corpuscular hemoglobin (picograms)	19.9–24.5	22.8	13.0–17.0	15.0
Mean corpuscular hemoglobin concentration (gm/dl)				
Wintrobe	31.0–34.0	33.0	31.0–35.0	33.0
Microhematocrit	32.0–36.0	34.0	30.0–36.0	33.2
Reticulocytes (%) (excludes punctate reticulocytes.)	0.0–1.5	0.8	0.2–1.6	0.6
Resistance to hypotonic saline (% saline solution producing) Minimum	0.40–0.50	0.46	0.66–0.72	0.69
Initial and complete hemolysis				
Maximum	0.32–0.42	0.33	0.46–0.54	0.50
Erythrocyte sedimentation rate	PCV 37	13%	PCV 35–40	7–27
(mm at 60 min)	PCV 50	0%		
RBC life span (days)	100–120		66–78	
RBC diameter (μm)	6.7–7.2	7.0	5.5–6.3	5.8

LEUKOCYTES	ADULT DOG	AVERAGE	ADULT CAT	AVERAGE
Leukocytes (per/μl)	6,000–17,000	11,500	5,500–19,500	12,500
Neutrophils—bands (%)	0–3	0.8	0–3	0.5
Neutrophils—mature (%)	60–77	70.0	35–75	59.0
Lymphocyte (%)	12–30	20.0	20–55	32.0
Monocyte (%)	3–10	5.2	1–4	3.0
Eosinophil (%)	2–10	4.0	2–12	5.5
Basophil (%)	Rare	0.0	Rare	0.0
Neutrophils—bands (per/μl)	0–300	70	0–300	100
Neutrophils—mature (per/μl)	3,000–11,500	7,000	2,500–12,500	7,500
Lymphocytes (no/μl)	1,000–4,800	2,800	1,500–7,000	4,000
Monocytes (no/μl)	150–1,350	750	0–850	350
Eosinophils (no/μl)	100–1,250	550	0–1,500	650
Basophils	Rare	0	Rare	0

*From Schalm, O. W., Tain, N. C., and Carroll, E. J.: Veterinary Hematology, 3rd ed. Philadelphia, Lea & Febiger, 1975.

APPENDIX 3

Canine Blood Values at Different Ages — Average Values*

AGE	RBC MILLIONS/μl	RETIC. %†	NUCL. RBC/ 100 WBC†	HB gm/dl
Birth	5.75	7.1	1.8	16.70
2 weeks	3.92	7.1	1.8	9.76
4 weeks	4.20	7.1	1.8	9.60
6 weeks	4.91	3.6	1.8	9.59
8 weeks	5.13	3.9	0.3	11.00
12 weeks	5.27	3.9	Rare	11.60

*From Andersen, A. C., and Gee, W.: Vet. Med., *53*:135, 1958.
†See Ewing, G. O., Schalm, O. W., and Smith, R. S.: J.A.V.M.A., *161*:1669, 1972.
Abbreviations: RBC, red blood cell; Retic., reticulocyte; Nucl, nucleated; Hb, hemoglobin; PCV, packed cell volume; WBC, white blood cell; Neut., neutrophil; Lymph, lymphocyte, Eos., eosinophil.

PCV VOL. %	WBC/μl	NEUT./μl	BANDS/μl	LYMPH./μl	EOS./μl
50	16,500	1,300	400	2,500	600
32	11,000	6,500	100	3,000	300
33	13,000	8,600	0	4,000	40
34	15,000	10,000	0	4,500	100
37	18,000	11,000	234	6,000	270
36	15,300	9,400	115	4,600	322

Canine Blood Values

BLOOD TEST MALE	WEANLING PUPPIES, MALES (6 WEEKS)			RAPID GROWTH PHASE MALES (12–24 Weeks)			
	5th Percentile	*Median*	*95th Percentile*	*5th Percentile*	*Median*	*95th Percentile*	
RBC ($\times 10^6/\mu l$)	3.33	3.88	4.49	4.71	5.32	6.03	
PCV (%)	22.2	26.9	32.6	30.9	36.4	42.0	
Hemoglobin (gm/dl)	7.4	8.6	10.2	11.1	12.8	14.9	
MCV (fl)	60	69	76	63	68	74	
WBC (no./μl)	7222	12100	17605	7770	12150	16340	
Bands (no./μl)	0	67	466	0	0	291	
Neutrophils (no./μl)	4766	7656	12582	4533	7590	11286	
Lymphocytes (no./μl)	1617	3615	6588	2009	3618	5754	
Monocytes (no./μl)	0	0	366	0	0	440	
Eosinophils (no./μl)	0	140	640	0	333	978	
Basophils (no./μl)	0	0	107	0	0	0	

BLOOD TEST FEMALE	WEANLING PUPPIES, MALE (6 WEEKS)			RAPID GROWTH PHASE FEMALES (12–24 WEEKS)			
	5th Percentile	*Median*	*95th Percentile*	*5th Percentile*	*Median*	*95th Percentile*	
RBC ($\times 10^6/\mu l$)	3.40	3.98	4.56	4.72	5.51	6.32	
PCV (%)	23.2	27.7	33.9	31.1	38.1	42.7	
Hemoglobin (gm/dl)	7.7	8.8	10.3	11.0	13.1	15.0	
MCV (fl)	61	70	76	63	68	74	
WBC (no./μl)	7908	12331	17360	7374	12200	18700	
Bands (no./μl)	0	0	433	0	95	390	
Neutrophils (no./μl)	4769	7726	13505	4370	7349	12469	
Lymphocytes (no./μl)	1706	3433	6462	2036	3839	5913	
Monocytes (no./μl)	0	0	334	0	105	445	
Eosinophils (no./μl)	0	128	630	0	335	932	
Basophils (no./μl)	0	0	166	0	0	0	

From D. F. Lawler, D. V.M.: Reference Intervals per Canine Blood Values. St. Louis, Ralston Purina Co., 1986.
5th percentile and 95th percentile: ranking indicates that 90 per cent of all values were between these points.
Median: One half of values were above this point, and one half were below.

	Young Adult Males (6–12 Months)			Adult Male Dogs (1 Year–11 Years)		
	5th Percentile	Median	95th Percentile	5th Percentile	Median	95th Percentile
	5.74	6.44	7.14	5.87	6.66	7.59
	39.0	44.5	50.3	41.1	48.2	55.0
	14.0	16.0	18.0	14.5	17.1	19.2
	65	69	74	66	71	79
	8314	12075	18623	6869	9509	13985
	0	0	234	0	0	212
	5043	7245	13416	4121	6745	10350
	1923	2943	5254	1108	2038	3303
	0	0	333	0	0	118
	38	663	2251	95	528	1749
	0	0	110	0	0	93

	Young Adult Females (6–12 Months)			Adult Female Dogs (1 Year–11 Years)		
	5th Percentile	Median	95th Percentile	5th Percentile	Median	95th Percentile
	5.67	6.61	7.23	5.61	6.60	7.46
	39.5	45.9	52.0	40.4	46.5	55.3
	14.8	16.6	18.3	14.2	16.6	18.9
	65	70	76	65	70	80
	7503	10825	15063	5939	10350	16650
	0	0	223	0	0	421
	4119	6882	10446	4424	7209	11706
	1638	2866	5308	1034	2193	4406
	0	0	298	0	0	402
	0	445	1859	0	582	1853
	0	0	105	0	0	50

Breeds

Siberian husky
Saint Bernard
Beagle
Doberman pinscher
Black and tan coonhound
Poodle
Miniature schnauzer
English setter
English pointer
German shepherd
Labrador retriever

APPENDIX 5

Feline Blood Values at Different Ages*

AGE	RBC MILLIONS/μl	HB gm/dl
Birth	4.95	12.2
2 weeks	4.76	9.7
5 weeks	5.84	8.4
Average†	4.80	7.5
Range†	3.90–5.70	6.6–8.4
6 weeks	6.75	9.0
8 weeks	7.10	9.4
Average†	5.90	7.5
Range	3.30–7.30	7.6–15.0

*From Schalm, O. W., Jain, N. C., and Carroll, E. J.: Veterinary Hematology, 3rd ed. Philadelphia, Lea & Febiger, 1975.
†See Anderson, L., Wilson, R., and Hay, D.: Res. Vet. Sci., 12:579, 1971.

PCV VOL. %	WBC/μl	NEUT./μl	LYMPH./μl
44.7	7,500		
31.1	8,080		
29.9	8,550		
26.2	11,770	4,600	6,970
21.0–33.5	7,500–14,500		4,500–9,400
35.4	8,420		
35.6	8,420		4,900
26.2	12,400	7,500	1,925–10,100
22–38	6,900–23,100		

Feline Blood Values

BLOOD TEST MALE	RAPID GROWTH PHASE (12–20 WEEKS) MALE			
	5th Percentile	**Median**	**95th** Percentile	
RBC ($\times 10^6/\mu l$)	5.64	6.99	8.11	
PCV (%)	26.9	33.5	40.2	
Hemoglobin (gm/dl)	8.4	10.4	12.8	
MCV (fl)	42	48	54	
	10th* Percentile	**Median**	**90th*** Percentile	
WBC (no./μl)	9985	16400	24430	
Bands (no./μl)	0	0	156	
Neutrophils (no./μl)	6339	11570	19879	
Lymphocytes (no./μl)	989	2925	6064	
Monocytes (no./μl)	0	0	292	
Eosinophils (no./μl)	352	851	1663	
Basophils (no./μl)	0	0	0	
BLOOD TEST FEMALE	RAPID GROWING PHASE (12–20 WEEKS) FEMALE			
	5th Percentile	**Median**	**95th** Percentile	
RBC ($\times 10^6/\mu l$)	5.71	6.85	8.27	
PCV (%)	27.4	32.8	39.3	
Hemoglobin (gm/dl)	8.6	10.5	12.9	
MCV (fl)	42	47	54	
	10th* Percentile	**Median**	**90th** Percentile	
WBC (no./μl)	8680	16050	28250	
Bands (no./μl)	0	0	0	
Neutrophils (no./μl)	5939	11199	22502	
Lymphocytes (no./μl)	921	2942	6193	
Monocytes (no./μl)	0	0	286	
Eosinophils (no./μl)	276	1007	1715	
Basophils (no./μl)	0	0	0	

Adapted from D. F. Lawler, D.V.M.: Reference Intervals for Feline Blood Values. St. Louis, Ralston Purina, Co., 1986.

5th percentile and 95th percentile: ranking indicates that 90 percent of all values were between these points.

Median: One half of values were above this point, and one half were below.

Data collected with domestic shorthair (American Shorthair) cats.

*Narrower interval reported as a result of wide range below 10th and above 90th percentiles.

YOUNG ADULT MALE (6–12 MONTHS)			ADULT MALE CATS (1 Year–13 Years)		
5th Percentile	Median	95th Percentile	5th Percentile	Median	95th Percentile
6.00	7.24	8.90	5.71	7.36	9.67
28.5	34.3	42.8	26.2	35.2	46.3
9.2	10.9	13.2	8.7	11.2	14.4
43	47	51	43	48	53
10th* Percentile	Median	90th* Percentile	10th* Percentile	Median	90*th Percentile
8689	16950	29020	6450	9985	19070
0	0	198	0	0	97
5521	10725	22595	3651	6947	13412
1855	3480	6938	1486	2785	4938
0	107	448	0	0	208
223	847	1816	211	533	1260
0	0	0	0	0	0

YOUNG ADULT FEMALE (6–12 Months)			ADULT FEMALE CATS (1 Year–13 Years)		
5th Percentile	Median	95th Percentile	5th Percentile	Median	95th Percentile
6.28	7.42	8.97	5.54	7.24	8.75
30.2	36.1	45.0	26.9	34.4	42.5
9.2	11.1	13.8	9.0	11.4	13.5
42	48	52	42	47	52
10th* Percentile	Median	90th* Percentile	10th Percentile	Median	90th* Percentile
8232	14600	25920	6728	10500	16905
0	0	199	0	0	114
5116	9997	19988	3842	6897	12201
1604	3048	5622	1055	2465	4647
0	33	313	0	68	329
229	850	1955	210	552	1454
0	0	0	0	0	5

Index

Note: Page numbers in *italics* indicate illustrations; those followed by t indicate tables; those in **boldface** denote procedures.